Dedication

This book is dedicated, first of all, to all my brothers and sisters of Turtle Island who must document their traditions in order to practice them. Religious freedom is guaranteed to almost everyone, except Native people. Those people living behind locked doors must fight for the right to pray our way. I offer you these written words to support that fight.

Second, this book is dedicated to all my brothers and sisters who have lost their traditions because of the forces of colonization. I hope these words help you find your way home.

Third, I dedicate this book to all persons in recovery, no matter what the color of your skin. We are all involved in a process of healing from what has been.

Fourth, this book is dedicated—out of respect for the elders, to my grandmother, and the old ones who have gone before—to the memory of the gentle way we once lived with Creation.

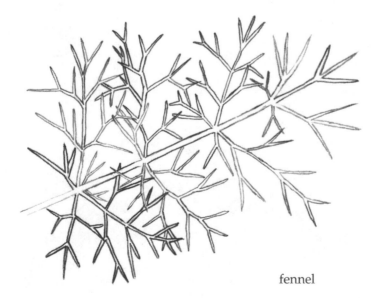

fennel

Sacred Smoke

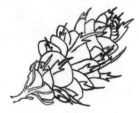

Sacred Smoke

the ancient art of smudging
for modern times

Harvest McCampbell

Native Voices
Summertown, Tennessee

Cover painting by Stan Padilla, *Yaqui*
Cover design by Warren Jefferson
Book design by Jerry Lee Hutchens
All plant illustrations by Ezra McCampbell, *Onondaga, Pawnee,* and
     Cheyenne
Other illustrations: John Kahionhes Fadden, *Akwesasne Mohawk,*
          pages 9 and 18; and Ken Rainbow Cougar Edwards, *Colville
          Confederated Tribes,* page 15.

Native Voices ☞

Book Publishing Company
P.O. Box 99
Summertown, TN 38483
1-888-260-8458
www.bookpubco.com

04 03 02 01   1 2 3 4

ISBN 1-57067-117-6

   McCampbell, Harvest, 1956-
      Sacred smoke : smudging, an ancient art for modern times /
   Harvest McCampbell.
         p. cm.
      Includes bibliographical references and index.
      ISBN 1-57067-117-6
      1. Smoke--Miscellanea. 2. Plants--Miscellanea.   I. Title.
   BF1623.I52M24 2002
   299'.74--dc21

   2002008946

Table of Contents

Acknowledgments

First of all I have a huge thank you for my son. He was always patient with my writing as a child. As a teenager he was my main editor on the first tiny versions of this book, and now as an adult he has demonstrated the awesome power of human resilience, worked on his own healing, and produced some of the artwork in this book. Son has been keeping me in firewood, tending the fire, and taking care of many other things so I can write.

Thank you Grandmother, for teaching me so much. I am definitely your child. Thanks to Josephine Peters and Ramona Duetschke as well as all the other elders who have taken the time to teach, correct, or encourage me.

Deep-felt appreciation goes to those who listened and supported me through that dark time when Son and I were both ill: Al Pierson, Patty and Allen Bayse, Richard Marshall, Cathy Metranga, Steven and Paola Barnhisel, Kevin Folley, Robyn Martin, Renee Shahrokh, Janice Barnes, Chris Partida, Josephine and Quetta Peters, Bonita Cowan, and Antonio Longwolf. I will pray Angels over your paths.

For encouragement, for their brazen sense of humor, for support and friendship above and beyond the call of duty, for their permanent presence in my life, I want to thank my buddies Judi Armbruster, Jana Noris, Sue Foust, Gen Corbin, Merty Moon, Diana DuEll, Robin Carneen, Lori Rigney, Mary McClelland, Cecilia Wyss, Terry Epp, Stephanie Ekcard, and Abena Songbird. Without your support and laughter, this little book might not have ever gotten done, and who knows if I would have even survived.

Two parts of this book were previously printed. "Suffering" was first published in *Pan Gia*, winter 1998-99. "Womens' Prayer" appeared in the *Circle Network News* newsletter, winter 1994-95.

Thanks are also due to Kirsten Freeman and Gianna Orozco of the Kim Yerton Memorial Library, for general encouragement and help with web sites and references. Last, but not least, a special acknowledgment goes to my ever patient and hopeful editor, Jerry Lee Hutchens.

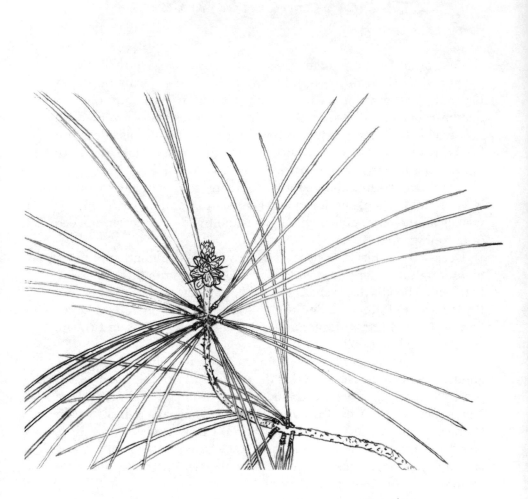

gray pine

A Spot in the Spiral

When I was a little girl Grandmother tried to teach me to say, "I am Iroquois Onondaga Oswegatchie, Bear Clan." There is very little that Grandmother tried to teach me that I refused. I refused to say these words. I was little. The words were big. What I heard in there that seemed familiar was the sound "dog." I knew I was not a dog. In that strange way of little children I refused to stretch my mouth around these words.

Grandmother settled on teaching me to say that I was Oswego, a shortened form of our band name. This is how I have referred to myself for most of my life. Our band is not federally recognized. So far as I know it is not organized. In fact, in my understanding, and as a result of doing some research, it appears that the United States government did a good job of dispersing the members long ago.

Most of my immediate family live in California, where I grew up. We are a long way from the place Grandmother's stories were born. When I was little I traveled with Grandmother, and saw firsthand how old teachings and knowledge were shared. The damaged bits of the web were repairing themselves before my eyes.

There was a fire that burned in Grandmother's heart. She followed the Ghost Dance religion and I was raised with its precepts in my heart. I offer you these words not as if I speak for a people, or from a certain tradition, but rather out of a vision that the damage done to the web of creation can be mended. That mending, that reweaving, is our real work.

Creation

First Woman was Grandmother Spider. She birthed herself from the void. It took a long time. A long, long time. It took eons of time. For she had nothing to work with except the power of her own thought. She dreamed her thought into substance, and as soon as she was born she began to spin.

She wove the sacred spiral upon which the universe was born. Stars hung like dew drops on a spider's web in the morn. As soon as she finished, she traveled back to the center, to the vortex, to the place where she was born, and she began to dance.

She took the sacred rattles and the four sacred bundles out of her pouch. She dreamed herself four daughters, one black, one red, one brown, one white. She placed one daughter on each bundle and danced and dreamed and thought them alive.

When they were fully alive, Grandmother Spider and her four daughters dreamed the Earth. When the Earth was finally ready, the daughters came to Earth to live. They became the mothers of the first human families and the sacred grandmothers of the four directions.

A long time passed. Grandmother Spider grew lonely for her children. She came to earth as Thought Woman. After wandering the earth she decided to make a home. She built her lodge in the forest near a meadow where a shaman and his apprentice lived.

She and the apprentice became lovers and together they had many children. Eventually, a drought came over the land and there was nothing to eat. Thought Woman's children were crying because they were hungry. She went to the shaman and his apprentice and said, "You must kill me so my children will not go hungry." At first they refused because they had both grown to love her.

She wandered around with tears in her eyes looking for something for her children to eat. When she was sure she could find nothing she insisted, "Kill me. It's the only way I'll ever be happy again."

When they finally agreed, she instructed them in how it was to be done. First they prepared a field by removing the rocks and larger plants. Then they used their digging sticks to rough up the surface of the soil. Next they cut Thought Woman's heart from her chest and planted it to the west of the field. Then they dragged her body across the field until all the flesh was worn from her bones. Last, they planted her bones to the east of the field.

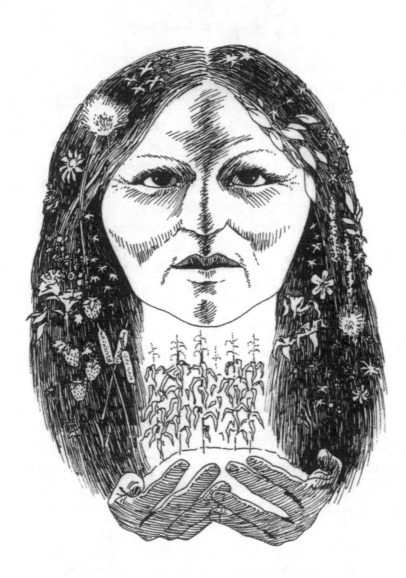

When they were finished, the Thunder Beings came to mourn her passing. Their tears make the land fertile, green and magic. From Thought Woman's heart grew the first oak tree. It had acorns of many kinds. From Thought Woman's flesh grew corn of many colors, and from Thought Woman's bones grew the sacred herbs for healing and ritual. These include the special sacred herbs to burn when we want her to hear our dreams.

Suffering

Grandmother took me to the woods. She showed me how everything is alive and full of Spirit. She showed me how everything communicated, even with a little tiny child. How even I could become part of it all, could become full with the beauty of the world.

The Sabbath school my mother dragged me to could never touch me. It was a dead place, full of dead people who could not communicate with Spirit. When you looked into their eyes there were no trees dancing in the wind, no stars dancing in their lazy spiral, no clouds hurrying on their journey across the sky. They did not know they could be part of it all. They were not full with the beauty of the world. There was nothing there that could touch me, nothing that left me with anything of value.

Except for their articulation of suffering. Ever since I was a tiny child I was fascinated with the suffering of little children who were to come unto Jesus. As I stood and listened to people argue its meaning, something began to grow inside me. Something began to awaken. I was horrified with the idea of suffering. I was fascinated with it. I knew, in that tiny child-like curious way, that there was something right and beautiful and true about the suffering that moves us towards something good and whole. And I knew that I was suffering in my tiny way, and that I would in a larger way dance with suffering and beauty as I moved towards what was good and whole all through my life.

I knew, because I had been in the woods. I had watched the suffering of one animal being devoured by another. I had watched the suffering of birth, of the little birds who worked so hard to feed their children. And I had my own suffering in that other world, that dead world. Suffering at the hand of my mother who was striving to erase everything alive from her soul. Striving to erase it because she could not stand the suffering of it all.

The Christians gave me that articulation of suffering. I listened, because my grandmother was no longer in this world. I had now to begin my own journey. I listened to the Christians until the knowing that was growing inside me was larger than their words. Then I found the Wiccans and I danced with them awhile, in their sweet naive circle that did not embrace suffering, and I caught a glance of that other circle, that dark circle, that arises when you don't embrace it all. Then I sat and listened to the Hindus speak of the suffering of the world, and the enlightened being's ability to rise above it, but I knew that for me, this was not the way to go. I listened to the Buddhists, I sat with the Zen masters. Then finally I came home to the woods.

The mosquito suffers in the dragonfly's jaws so that there will always be dragonflies. The dragonfly suffers in the little bird's beak so there will always be little birds. The little bird suffers in the hawk's talons so there will always be hawks. I suffer the bite of the mosquito, so that there will always be dragonflies and little birds and hawks.

My grandmother suffered that I may weave baskets, gather medicine, sit quietly, full of the beauty of the world. My mother suffered, for she would rather have given up the child who reminded her that she was rejected because she was red. And she suffered more when I turned out blue eyed, and for a while, blonde haired, and Grandmother raised me red anyway. And my aunties suffered when my grandmother neglected their children to take me to the woods, to teach me to weave. And I have suffered for my redness, for my blue eyes. And those who came before my grandmother suffered in ways I can only imagine. But I take my place in the circle, and through the gift of all of this suffering I have something to share.

I watch with pride as my son who suffered through it all with me takes his place in the circle of the sweat lodge, in the circle of the drum, in the circle of the round house, in the circle of prayer. In pride I watch as he takes his place in the circle of that other world, and through his suffering gives it something full of life.

Today I sit quietly with a Dineh child, with a young boy, and we weave a basket. Today there are many new basket weavers. And each waits for my help. But this one small child's is the one that matters the most. He is suffering with this basket. He cannot make it go right. His friends repeatedly run by, asking him to come play. But he knows something in that tiny child-like curious way. He knows something about hawks and mosquitoes. So he stays and struggles quietly with his basket. Follows me as I make the rounds of new basket weavers, sits with me when I sit.

Finally, he finds the star's lazy spiral dance. Finally he pulls it into a circle. This is all that really matters. I was taught that healing is about pulling the circle out of the chaos. And he has done it. He beams, he is like a tiny quiet star beside me.

And my son, as a teenager, gifted me with his first finished basket, and here in the circle of this Sacred valley, he has helped many others struggle with their first baskets. And I look all around me, and there are circles in many hands, baskets to remember the Old Ones by. Circles out of chaos. And I too beam, a tiny quiet tired star, full of the beauty and the suffering, full of the many circles all reflecting the one Sacred Circle.

This is our way. We do not rise above the suffering. We do not turn our eyes away. We embrace it prayerfully. In the heat of the sweat lodge. At the end of Sun Dance tethers. In the way we live our lives. We embrace suffering. We dance with suffering, and through suffering we pull the circle out of the chaos and continue to move towards what is beautiful and good and whole.

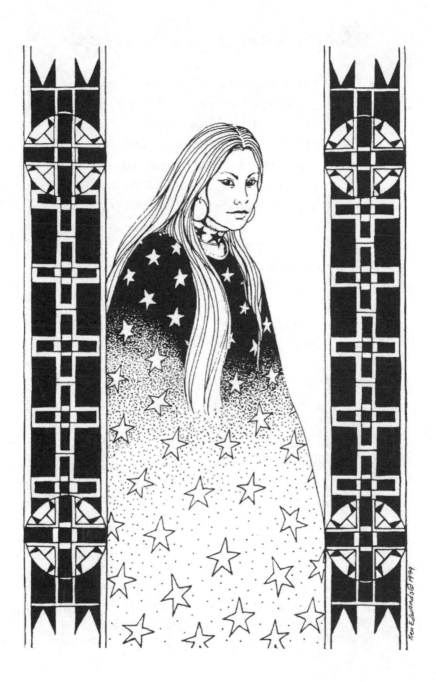

Women's Prayer

Grandmothers, we stand before you, behold us.
Powers of the East, behold us.
First quarter Moon, behold us.
Plant People, who gift us colorful dyes, behold us.
Rainbow Woman, inspire us,
as we learn to express outward.
Pine smudge, purify us, as we begin our journey.

Daughters, we stand before you, behold us.
Powers of the South, behold us.
Full Moon, behold us.
Plant People, who gift us food, behold us.
Corn Woman, nurture us, as we learn to nurture outward.
Mullein smudge, protect us, as we continue our journey.

Granddaughters, we stand before you, behold us.
Powers of the West, behold us.
Last quarter Moon, behold us.
Plant People, who gift us vision, behold us.
Crazy Woman, inspire us, as we learn to express inward.
Mugwort smudge, guide us, as we continue our journey.

Sisters, we stand before you, behold us.
Powers of the North, behold us.
New Moon, behold us.
Plant People, who gift us caution, behold us.
Death Woman, nurture us, as we learn to nurture inward.
Cedar smudge, consecrate our hearts,
as we complete our journey.

Sacred Smoke

Smudging

The burning of herbs or incense is a Sacred practice held in common by many traditions. In American Indian traditions we call this practice "smudging" or sometimes "smoking," even though the herbs may not be inhaled.

Smudging, practiced traditionally, takes many forms. Sometimes we tie the herbs in a bundle called a "smudge stick" and allow them to dry. There are some herbs that lend themselves to braiding, such as the sweet grass that you may have noticed in the movie "Dances With Wolves." In the Old Way, the end of the smudge stick or braid was lit from the council, central, or cooking fire. Now we often use a candle. Matches aren't very efficient because it takes a while to get the stick smoking.

In some cultures, pinches or even branches of herbs are placed directly in a camp or council fire, or onto the burning wood in an indoor fireplace.

In other cultures, a coal is removed from the fire and placed in a special receptacle. The Sacred herbs (which are hung to dry and then crumbled) are sprinkled on the hot coal. Today some people use prepared, quick-lighting charcoal. It's available from many Indian trading posts, at powwows, health-food stores, new age shops, and even Bible and Christian supply stores. Smudging is similar to Catholic and Orthodox incense burning, for which Bible and Christian supply stores carry prepared charcoal.

The container used as a receptacle for your lighted charcoal and Sacred herbs needs to be fireproof. Ceramic and glass bowls or abalone shells work well. There are also special chalices designed for smudging. Unless you use a chalice, place a layer of soil, sand, or salt in the bottom for insulation before adding your charcoal and herbs. The charcoal and smoldering herbs can heat the container up enough to scorch the surface it's resting on or the hand holding it.

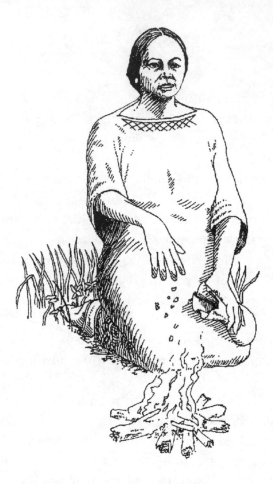

If you prefer to light your whole bundle or braid, hold it in a candle flame until the smudge glows red. Blow out the flame; it should smolder at least a few minutes. You'll need a bowl or shell to catch the hot ashes.

When burning bundles or braids of smudge, they will eventually go out themselves. Should you need to put them out before they do, you can easily tamp them out as you would a cigarette or cigar. If you are burning herbs in a special receptacle, you can use a stick or spoon to gently tamp out the charcoal and herbs. The addition of a small amount of water also will do the trick if you are in a hurry. Using water is messier and is considered, in some cultures, disrespectful to the Fire Spirits.

There are many Indian tribes, each with their own culture and belief systems. Not all tribes view the smoke rising from the herbs in the same light. And different herbs may be used for different purposes, depending on the person's tribe of origin. Speak with your family elders or do research at university libraries or regional museums to uncover clues about how your ancestors used herbs in prayer.

Commonly at powwows and other public events, sage, sweet grass and/or cedar are burned to purify one's self, one's space, and one's spiritual or healing tools. After lighting the smudge, we offer it to the cardinal directions, or hold it near our hearts. We wash or fan the smoke over our bodies by first bringing it towards the heart, then inhaling, pulling it up over the head, washing it down the arms, etc.

We also burn herbs during healing work and prayer. This helps one connect to one's higher power. The smoke carries one's intention to the Sky World, where the Spirit Beings and our ancestors live.

During healing work, the smoke may be directed over the patient by blowing, or fanning either with the hand or with feathers. This clears out old unhealthy energy and brings in the special attributes of the herbs.

Gathering Plants for Smudge

In the old days there were tribal and family rules and teachings on gathering herbs. Many of these rules are still in effect. Some of these old rules have been incorporated into tribal resource management laws. In a few places the old rules may be nearly forgotten.

These old rules and teachings existed for the purpose of protecting and allocating resources. They defined who may collect, where they had rights to collect, and when and how this collecting was to be done.

These old rules also embraced the idea of the collector as having a responsibility towards the plants and landscapes utilized as resources. Native people were born with responsibilities for the natural world. The housewife, herbalist, hunter, and healer all had the responsibility for tending the environments they drew their sustenance from. (Read *Ceremony* by Leslie Marmon Silko for more on this concept. There is a healer herbalist character in the book who embodies this concept of tending the natural world.)

There is great diversity in how tribes and families approach and resolve these issues. This information can often be uncovered by speaking with elders or research in archives of museums and university libraries.

Today, not only must we strive to respect the old rules of our ancestors and the ancestors of the land we inhabit, we must also be aware of modern laws. Today it is actually unlawful to gather herbs in much of North America. Depending on where and how those laws are broken, the result can be as mild as a stern lecture or as costly as a $25,000 fine and possible jail time.

Get the facts before you collect. Collecting on private land is generally acceptable, as long as you have written permission from the property owner and are not disturbing endangered species. Gathering herbs on any land designated as a park, parkway, or monument is generally unlawful. Special permits can sometimes be obtained by Native people for cultural use. Contact the local administration of the public land in question for more information.

Gathering on Bureau of Land Management or Forest Service land is generally acceptable with permission. Check out a map of the area you wish to collect in to see whose jurisdiction that land falls under. Call the administration office for the area from which you wish to collect. They will ask you how much of what kinds of plant material you plan to harvest. They will probably ask you how you will be collecting the material. Generally they want to know if you will be removing whole plants or if you will be disturbing the soil in any way. They also want to know if you will be leaving any plant parts behind, such as when a tree is chopped down and its limbs are left behind.

If you are gathering a small amount of material for personal or cultural use and you do not plan to sell the results of your endeavors, remove whole plants, disturb the soil or leave a mess—then verbal permission may be all you need. In this case make sure you write down the person's name giving the permission and their phone number. Carry this information with you when you gather, in case you are stopped. I have had to prove I had permission on more than one occasion.

You may be required to get a permit in certain situations. Be sure you carry any required permits with you when gathering.

Gathering on Indian reservations is controlled by tribal law. Generally only tribal members of the specific reservation in question may gather on that reservation. Additional rules may also be in force. Breaking these laws is the same as breaking any other governmental agency's laws. Fines and jail time can be incurred.

As you can well imagine, all of this provides a certain level of difficulty to Native people trying to practice their culture. This situation prevails whether we are talking about gathering herbs, basket materials, or other items used in arts and in the production of utilitarian objects. It also has a huge effect on traditional food practices for many people.

Considering all of this makes it even more important to respect the old rules, as the resources are less available for the people's use than they were in the old days.

I want to share with you some of Grandmother's rules. You can follow these rules, in addition to the modern laws, until you are taught the proper rules for your people and for the land where you live.

We always prayed before we gathered. We brought offerings for the plants and the spirits. This was often tobacco and corn meal. We always spoke to the plants and asked their permission to gather. We told the plants what our purpose was and thanked them if we were allowed to gather.

Grandmother also taught me to always leave enough for the next year and the next family. (The next family might not be human; animals have a right to subsistence too.) Each plant or stand of plants has the right to reproduce. We never took the only flower. If there was only one of a particular plant, we never took more than a leaf or two.

It was important to Grandmother to gather in such a way that the casual observer would not notice the plant had been collected from. She also liked to do her gathering in prayerful solitude, away from curious onlookers.

Other good rules I have heard are never to gather from more than 30% of the plants in a stand and never to take more than 30% from the plants that you do collect from. I have also heard that in some traditions you do not gather from the Grandparent plant, nor from the youngest offspring.

All of these ways of thinking about gathering help protect the resource. I tend to keep each of them in mind when I gather. I take the time before I start to carefully observe the plants. I want to get a feeling for the elder plant among them, and also determine which are the youngest and most fragile. I want to do my collecting in a way that tends the plants, that contributes to their health and strength rather than in a way that creates weakness and disease. I also think about who else may use these plants and take only my fair share.

I believe every plant has a right to reproduce. I keep this in mind when I gather. If I must use roots, I try to dig after the plant has gone to seed, and leave the seeds behind. If the plant will regrow from its crown or a piece of root, I make sure to leave that behind in a place it will be likely to grow.

Also the cleaner the air, the less exposed to pesticides and other toxins, the better. In today's world we need to be reasonable in our expectations, but careful enough not to poison ourselves.

In addition to these general considerations, you will also find some specific considerations for the individual plants listed under gathering tips in the sections on herbs.

For more thoughts on tending the patches where you gather check out http://www.trinityalpsbotanicals.com. They have a page devoted to thoughts on gathering listed under "Wildcrafting Guidelines." The book *Native Plants Native Healing* by Tis Mal Crow also has some very useful and thought-provoking information on gathering wild plants in the introduction and first chapters of the book.

Moon Time

There are many cultural taboos on gathering herbs. In most traditions when a woman is on her moon, she may not gather, or in some cases even touch the plant medicines. But in a few cultures the particular power of a woman on her moon is considered beneficial for the preparation of particular herbal and ceremonial items.

The safe rule is to abstain from gathering or preparing smudge and other medicines during moon time, unless you are taught differently by your own elders. If you are taught differently, it is still a good idea to remember that every tradition is not the same, and keep your moon medicines separate from those that may be used in an intertribal way.

It is also a good idea not to touch any smudge or other ceremonial items or regalia when you are on your moon, unless you are taught differently within a specific culture. Women should not use the sweatlodge when they are on their moon. They must stay away from the drum, out of the circle, away from most ceremonial houses, and away from those preparing for ceremony. Not following these taboos causes sickness to the woman and those attending, participating, and observing.

Moon time is a woman's time to care for herself. It is a time of inward reflection, meditation, and personal rebirth. Most Native traditions honored women by allowing her this time. In the modern work-a-day world, we often do not get the chance to rest and reflect and that is why this time is often accompanied by imbalance.

Moon time is considered a very powerful force in many traditions—so powerful that in some traditions girls may not gather medicines until after they become women. And they can no longer gather after they become elders and no longer cycle with the moon. However, these cultures almost always follow the taboos against gathering or preparing smudge and other plant medicines while a woman is on her moon.

Seek time with your elders, they are your best teachers. If no one alive remembers, search out ethnographic materials in museums and university libraries. Very often there are recorded or microfiched materials archived away but available for public research.

Making Smudge Sticks

I once heard an elder say, "There is a ceremony before the ceremony, and there are ceremonies within the ceremony, and then there are ceremonies after the ceremony is complete." He was speaking about powwows. But he could have been talking about making smudge.

I am sharing this with you because I am trying to get at some deep thoughts, deep thoughts on the traditions around making smudge. I could tell you exactly how I do it, and symbolically what all that means to me, but that would probably be doing you a disservice.

The symbol systems and the deep stories I grew up with are probably very different from yours. It is important to know that each step and the steps before and after are all important. These are things you should seek guidance on from your family elders, the elders of your own traditions.

I am going to share with you some of the things I have been taught about making smudge. I am doing this to feed your thoughts and give you questions for your elders, and not as rules for how things should be done.

Before gathering herbs, most people pray. Some people bathe in a specially prepared ritual bath, or they smudge, sweat, abstain from eating meat, or even fast. I pray. I ask for guidance or permission and wait to feel the presence of that guidance. And I never gather for others when I am in pain or ill in any way.

I was also taught to ask the plant's permission. If you were not raised within the traditions of Native religion this may seem like a strange thing to do. I have taught people to try to remember back when they were children. Sometime back when each of us were tiny we knew how to talk to plants and to spirits. When we tried to talk to adults about this we might have been told we had a "wild imagination," that we told "tall tales," or something else to the same effect.

If you can remember the words that were used to label your connection with Spirit as something other than right and natural you can probably get in touch with the part of yourself that was born knowing how to communicate with plants. Tell yourself "I am going to imagine what it feels like to ask this plant's permission." You can replace "imagine" with whatever the potent word is for you. I know this sounds silly, but it really works.

I have been taught to cut or snap the herbs from the plant in the exact length that I am going to use them, and as soon as they are cut to hang them upside down so the energy does not drain out. When I am bundling the herbs I have been taught to have all the stems at one end so the parts of the plants that were closest to the earth are all together. I was taught that within the smudge bundle the plants are still symbolically expressing their connection to the earth through their cut stems being bundled together.

I was taught that plants, when growing, express the movement of prayer. This movement is from the Earth to the Sky World where the ancestors and the Creator dwell. When making smudge with this symbol system in mind, it is important that the growing tips of the plants are all at the same end of the smudge stick so the energy is all moving in this symbolic direction from earth to sky.

The way I was taught, it is very important not to bend or fold the herbs. This interferes with the symbolic movement of energy. It is also important not to trim the growing tips, this symbolically lets the energy out and trims back one's connection to the sky.

When the smudge bundle is wrapped with the string that holds it together, I was again taught to think of prayer and the movement of prayer. I was also taught to think of the moment of creation and the sacred spiral. The string spirals up the smudge stick from the cut ends to the growing tips from earth to sky, and then back down from sky to earth. This is the symbolic movement of prayer and creation. I was taught that prayer and creation are ongoing dynamic interrelated processes.

Your traditions may be very different. I hope you will seek out knowledgeable elders so that you can keep your own traditions alive.

Now for a few mundane notes on making smudge: I have found that it is helpful to allow the herbs to wilt for a few hours or a few days, depending on the time of year and the herbs used. This should be done inside or in the shade. Provision can be made during the wilting process for the cut stems to be above the tips to keep the energy from draining out.

Your intention here is to allow some of the moisture content to evaporate and for the plants to become a bit limp, making them easier to bundle. This reduced moisture content will also help prevent mildew and mold. It will take a bit of practice to find just the right amount of wilt. You do not want your plants to become so dry that they become brittle.

Next when you are wrapping your bundles, wrap them firmly but not tightly. This will also take a bit of practice to find just the right touch. Bundles that are wrapped too tightly may mold or mildew. If this happens the bundles should not be used.

Bundles that are wrapped too tightly will not burn properly because they will not be able to breathe. On the other hand, bundles that are wrapped too loosely may fall apart, dropping glowing coals. I once received a very painful burn in this way.

You might want to form a little string loop on the stem end when wrapping your smudge so the bundle can continue drying hanging with the stem ends up. They can be allowed to finish drying indoors away from the moist night air. Hanging by the loop is a nice way to store them until they are used. However, if they are to be stored for a long period of time an earthenware crock, cedar chest, or other similar container will help keep them fresh by preventing all the essential oils from evaporating.

I like to use unbleached 100% cotton crochet string, organically grown when available. Synthetic string can release toxins when burned. Animal hair fibers do not smell pleasant when burned. Hand spun plant fibers were probably the original binding materials for smudge bundles, making them very time-consuming, labor-intensive, and valuable to our ancestors.

Plant Names

All of the plants included in this book have many names. They have Native names and familiar nicknames. They have English language common names sometimes particular to small regions, and they have botanical names. Each of these systems of naming and classifying reflects how the culture doing the naming thinks of plants.

In Native and traditional cultures plants are named and classified in a way that defines something about that plant's spirit, energy, appearance, habits, or its uses.

In scientific circles plants are classified by minute details of their structure and by genetics. Scientific or botanical names are given by the scientist or explorer who "discovered" them, or who convinced other scientists that this particular set of structural or genetic variations deserves its own name. Sometimes these plants are named for the wife, mistress, or secretary of the "discovering" person, if not actually named for this person. Sometimes they are given Latin names that actually describe something significant about the plant.

I have tried to use names that will enable you to find more information about these plants. I have certain habits in the names I use for these plants. If I were speaking to you I might use different names. But here, I have tried to use accessible names so you can learn more, and be certain of your identification.

Correctly identifying a plant by botanical name will give you the greatest access to information on its uses, history, and any possible toxicity.

Most Native systems of defining, classifying, naming, and using plants do not resemble scientific or botanical practice. However, until you have an experienced teacher who has used the plants over many years, I hope you will pay close attention to scientific identification.

Ritual

Ritual is any action undertaken with intention and belief that grows powerful through repetition and connection. The repetition can be personal, through this lifetime or many lifetimes. It can be cultural, such as tooth brushing after every meal. Or it can be ancestral, such as the autumn dances held throughout California by the Indians who have lived here for thousands of years.

Finding one's own personal ritual is a very healing experience. All rituals have a beginning point. Many traditional rituals began as dreams or visions. Often the ritual evolved out of the enactment of the dream or vision. Direct instruction for ritual sometimes came from Spirit helpers. This still happens today. It is possible that Spirit will instruct you through dreams or visions if you ask and open your heart.

Another way rituals evolve is by paying attention to one's feelings as one makes or attempts to make Sacred or Healing actions. The right actions feel good. A sense of well-being and connection, of magic, creeps into one's soul. Some people experience this quickly, but for others it evolves slowly. Patience and commitment are required as with any new endeavor.

Personal herbal rituals can evolve out of brewing tea or burning herbs. You can research how your genetic or spiritual ancestors used herbs. You can ask your family elders about various practices used in the past. You can read or take classes, using information while watching your feelings.

I gather herbs in a Sacred Way, with my intention made known to the plant, or following the plant's instruction to me. This act alone weaves me into the web of life and the universe. It connects me to both my ancestors and to all people and beings who have lived in a Sacred Way.

The ritual of gathering herbs in a Sacred Way is powerful healing for my soul. The time I spend with the Plant People sustains me through computer time and cement jungle time.

When you find your right and perfect ritual, I know it will sustain you too. Let the searching flow through your heart, let it be spontaneous. There is no exact recipe for your personal healing rituals, but with patience and commitment I know you will find them.

Reclaiming Tradition

I would like to offer a few words of comfort and advice to those who think their traditions have been lost.

One of my teachers once said, "Harvest, nothing can be lost, because it was all dreamed to begin with. It can be dreamed again. At the heart of creation, time does not exist."

This thought is a great comfort to me. I hope it will comfort you also. However, it does not mean that you should just go out and dream up any old thing and call it tradition.

Native tradition has always existed on a continuum. The old ones teach the young ones, person to person. Native tradition has also always existed in the context of community, where certain values, beliefs, and practices are held in common.

Reading this book may be a part of your journey to reclaim some of your tradition. But it can only be a part of that journey. Seek the teachings of your old ones, even if you must seek their words in archived collections of universities or museums. There is probably a record somewhere of the tribe or band-specific information you need.

If there are living elders to your tradition, arrange your life so you have time to sit at their knee. It is the greatest gift you can ever give yourself. Find some way to be of service to their concerns and endeavors. Don't expect immediate acceptance.

I spent seven years "courting" an elder who is very important to me. At first she mostly ignored me, and was at times a bit rude. But I just kept being there, treating her with respect, listening to her every word, and bringing her little gifts of medicine plants from many cultures.

Eventually we became close friends and I had the opportunity to sit at her knee full-time for about nine months. That truly was the greatest gift I ever gave myself, the greatest gift I ever received.

Learning about tradition is not something to undertake lightly or to think of as anything less than a lifetime journey.

Words of Caution

I would like to encourage you to invite herbs into your life. But do so with caution and respect. Read everything you can find on the herbs you are interested in and pay attention, not only to their beneficial effects, but also to any potential side effects. Listen to your inner voice. Given the chance, it may prove itself to be infinitely wise.

As you explore you will gain research skills to supplement your intuition and inner voice. Rather than blindly following your herbalist's or a salesperson's advice, use your new skills. Don't allow someone else's misinformation or forgetfulness to cause you potential harm.

Before using any plant, make sure you have not confused it with something toxic or harmful. Growing your own is the safest practice for those who do not have a teacher to study with.

Smoke from herbs can cause allergic reactions, or trigger asthma and other respiratory distress. The information in this book is offered for its historical and cultural value. Neither the author nor the publisher assumes any responsibility for the way in which any individual responds to the smoke from any herbs. The information contained in this book is not intended to be used as a substitute for medical advice, diagnosis, or treatment. If you choose to burn herbs, please use common sense and moderation. Discontinue use and see your doctor if any irritation develops.

Never leave burning smudge, charcoal, candles, or fires unattended. Never use smudge around flammable substances. The main idea behind burning herbs is to release their energy and fragrance, not to fill your room or your lungs with smoke. Burning excessive amounts of smudge or burning smudge too often can lead to respiratory distress and other respiratory problems. A curl or two of smoke rising from your herbs is all that is necessary. If your eyes are burning or you're coughing or suppressing the urge to cough, you're either using herbs that don't agree with you or making way too much smoke. (Put out smudge, open the windows, leave the room, and close the door.)

Show consideration for other people when burning smudge. Everyone except traditional medicine people should avoid burning smudge in the same room as infants, anyone who is pregnant, those suffering from respiratory problems, or those who have asthma or respiratory allergies.

To avoid fire hazards, never use smudge around flammable substances. Never leave burning smudge, charcoal, candles, or fires unattended.

Pregnancy

Pregnancy is not a good time to begin experimenting with smudge. Most of the herbs can cause miscarriage in people whose bodies are not familiar with their use. If you become pregnant, consider moderating or stopping your use of smudge. Avoid inhaling smudge smoke directly or avoid it entirely. If you are having trouble getting pregnant, you might want to avoid smudging for a few months just in case it may help.

My Favorite Herbs for Smudge

All the herbs included in this book are personally familiar to me. I have held them in my hands and used them for prayer and healing. These plants are medicine. They are not harmless and must be used with respect for their power. Don't forget to have this attitude of respect towards the power of these healing plants.

Some of the herbs I have included are found in both North America and around the globe. For one of these herbs, fennel, I primarily discuss its European history. This herb is used in Native healing in a different context than is being discussed here.

The herbs included are those which you might be exposed to at a powwow or other event where the public is welcome. I have not included anything secret or private. I have not included anything that I feel is really none of my or the public's business because it is only used in specific, private, tribal ceremonies. And I have not included any plants that are not already available for purchase.

As you read, listen for the whisperings of the grandmothers in between the lines. As you learn, spend time in nature with the living plants in many seasons. Really notice them. Sit quietly and listen, breathe, watch. Plants have a secret life that does not reveal itself to the hurried observer.

Gather the medicines and pray. Remember the best teacher is an experienced elder, and not a book. It is that humble respect for the experienced elder that will most fully bring the medicine alive.

Bayberry

(*Myrica*, various species)
Also called Waxberry, Wax Myrtle,
Sweet Fern, and Sweet Gale

bayberry

Bayberry, or sweet fern, leaves are used as a religious incense, much as either sage or sweet grass. The leaves are dried, sometimes bundled together, other times left loose or crumbled. The fragrance is warm, sweet, and pungent. In some traditions, it is the preferred herb for making offerings and as an addition to the water used in the sweat lodge.

When I was growing up I would travel with Grandmother from California's Central Valley to the mountains near the Mendocino coast to gather bayberries and bayberry leaves. Bayberry and its close relatives can be found in many parts of the coastal mountains along both the Pacific and Atlantic oceans.

Grandmother used the bayberries to make candles. She would steep dried bayberries in slowly heating paraffin. After the paraffin had taken on the scent and a bit of the color of the bayberries, she would strain the berries out and pour the paraffin into a candle mold, with the wick weighted in place. The wick was often tied around a pencil or small stick, which rested across the top of the mold. A metal washer was tied to the bottom of the wick to ensure it stayed in place. After the wax set she removed the candles from their molds, usually small coffee cans. She would warm up the previously strained waxy berries and apply them to the outside of the candles. Sometimes she added more berries and a final extra layer of wax. These candles were given as special gifts, and we burned one each night during our evening prayers. I clearly remember the lovely scent.

Other uses: Grandmother used the leaves to make tea for fever and upset stomach. This pleasant tea relieved many of my childhood miseries. I have had occasion to use them this way myself. The tea has as pleasant a taste as the berries' scent, making it a very agreeable remedy. The root bark, which I have never used, is reported to be useful for diarrhea and hemorrhage and also useful as a gargle for sore throats.

The wax from the berries can be used in soap making. The berries and leaves can be used in potpourri and other crafts. The leaves and berries can be used for dye, producing various colors depending on the mordant.

Bayberry leaves are known to repel insects. A few added to containers of flour and other dry goods may reduce the incidence of food pests and moths in your kitchen cupboards. Their pleasant taste will make them a nice addition to a pot of winter tea or a jar of summer sun-infused tea. It is not important to use them sparingly, and an occasional cup of tea made from them just for the pleasure of it is perfectly fine.

Growing tips: Bayberry shrubs make a nice addition to the home landscape, especially for people who like surprises. They are such a variable group of plants that you might not be sure exactly what the young plant you bring home will grow up to be.

In maturity most specimens, including Eastern bayberry (*Myrica pennsylvania*) and Western bayberry (*Myrica californica*) will reach 10-15 feet. There are dwarf varieties of *Myrica pusilla* and *Myrica cerifera* as small as 1-3 feet. And there are varieties of all these species that sometimes reach up to 30 feet in height. Make sure your supplier provides height information before you choose your plants. And then be prepared to be surprised.

Bayberry also has varieties that are evergreen (*Myrica californica*), however a few lose their leaves in winter. One of these deciduous varieties puts on a fall show by turning maroon before dropping its leaves. There are, however, strains of *Myrica pennsylvania* which retain their leaves through the winter. Read the descriptions in your plant catalogs, or purchase locally, in the fall, when you can see for yourself if the leaves are turning colors.

The leaves of *Myrica pennsylvania* are narrow and leathery. Those of *Myrica californica* look a bit as if someone took a pair of pinking shears to their edges. Other species have edges that appear slightly turned under. The leaves on all varieties are a glossy dark green color, sometimes almost a blue-green. The undersides of the leaves are much lighter in color and the veins appear raised.

Berries are found on female plants only. However, if you grow your own you will need to plant both male and female plants to be sure to get berries. Have a conversation with your plant supplier about the particular need of the varieties you purchase. Make sure you let them know whether or not you want berries.

Generally the shrubs will do best in partial sun to bright filtered shade with fairly good drainage. They will be happiest with some coastal influence, however, with a little effort and irrigation they can thrive away from the coast and in full sun. Once established the plants are drought-tolerant.

One species will thrive in boggy or moist soils: *Myrica gale*, which is normally a small shrub from 2-6 feet. *Myrica gale* produces resinous nutlets rather than actual berries.

All varieties can be shorn to form hedges, allowed to grow naturally as specimens or screens, or grown in a container and trained to the shape of a small tree.

Gathering tips: When your bayberry plants are mature, or when gathering from the wild, here are a few instructions to help the plants stay healthy. When picking the berries gently hold the branch with one hand, and gently massage the berries off with the other. The mature leaves growing back away from the tip of the branches are the preferred ones to gather. Be careful when collecting them to not break the branch or strip the bark. Using both hands is best. This way you can protect the twigs from breaking. A little practice will teach you how to best remove the leaves without stripping the bark.

California Bay

(*Umbellularia californica*)
Also called Pepperwood, Oregon Myrtle, and Myrtle Wood

My first experience with California bay as a smudge was in 1990. A friend and I were in the mountains gathering herbs in a Sacred Way. I observed him in conversation with a bay tree. I was surprised at their agreement on the amount of leaves to be gifted and accepted. Later, I asked what he was going to do with all the bay leaves. "I'm going to use them for smudge." I didn't think that was traditional, and told him so. He didn't care what I thought. It was between him and the bay.

As it turned out, within a few days, I accidentally ran across a reference to California Indians' historic use of bay leaf smudge in the autumn to protect against colds and flu! At the time I lived in central California, and was not aware of bay or pepperwood leaves being used as a smudge, even though I was very familiar with their use as a medicine.

I now live in northern California. Here pepperwood leaves are often used to create smoke. The leaves are burned to clean sweat lodges before and after use. They are used in a similar fashion during certain other ceremonies. The leaves are sometimes used as offerings to the fire at sweat lodges and other ceremonial fires. This offering may be made as part of a prayer, to make "medicine," or as food for the fire. Additionally, a few bay leaves are sometimes added to the water bucket that is used for sprinkling on the rocks and drinking during sweats.

Other uses: Bay leaves are sometimes stored with regalia and baskets to discourage insects. They should be dried first and care must be taken that they do not stain valuable material. One or two dried bay leaves can also be added to containers of flour, rice, etc. to discourage pests. They will impart a very subtle fragrance to the

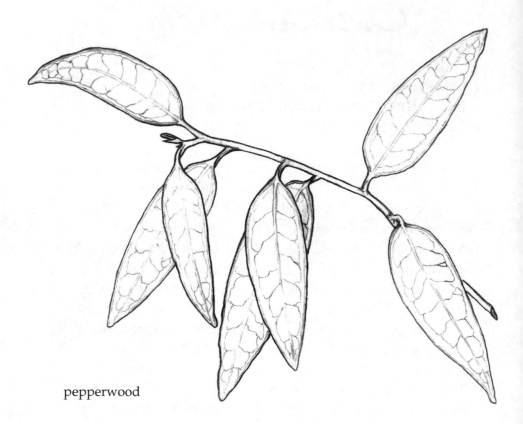

pepperwood

foods they are stored with. This fragrance usually does not last after cooking.

One or two bay leaves are also put in water on or near the wood stove or over the pilot light of a gas stove as a type of "aromatherapy" for colds and flu.

Modern interpretation of traditional uses of bay leaves include infusing the leaves in oil for chest and muscle rubs and extracting then in glycerine with other herbs for cough syrup. Bay cannot withstand high temperatures for long. The heat will drive off all the essential oils. Remember, they should only be used in moderation internally.

Bay leaves have traditionally been used in cooking. Used sparingly, they add a unique and subtle flavor to foods. I use a leaf or two in soups and gravies. I sometimes place a leaf in the bottom of a baking pan when making cake, sweet dessert, or breakfast foods. Last, but not least, one or two bay leaves can be added to a pot of beans at the beginning of cooking to flavor them, improve digestibility, and reduce toot.

Bay leaves are also sometimes added to potpourri, and are used in making wreaths and other crafts.

Another part of the bay commonly used are the "peppernuts." The outer fleshy covering, when fresh, and the grated nuts are used as a poultice to draw out poison. Traditional applications include spider, insect, and other minor bites; festering splinters, stickers, and other minor infections; impetigo; and warts.

The outer coverings were once prepared as a dessert, but I don't know how. The nuts are roasted and eaten sparingly or ground and brewed similar to coffee, with a similar but more powerful effect. I haven't tried it, but I have been told that two or three nuts give a lift that lasts all day.

Growing tips: California bay can be grown in filtered shade in cool moist areas and in full shade with irrigation in hotter, inland climates. With cool moist coastal influences it will often tolerate full sun. In desert environments it will need to be grown in a container on a protected porch or a bright spot in the house. Bay loves moisture, yet it needs good drainage. Often bay is found in acid soils. The trees can reach up to 100 feet tall in favorable conditions. Some forest specimens have branches that sprawl along the ground and then lift up to the sun with a total spread of up to 100 feet. Your bay tree is most likely to reach 20-30 feet with an equal spread. Keep this in mind when planting. Make sure you look up and watch out for power lines. If grown near structures your bay tree will need periodic pruning and thinning. In the wild, they sometimes become top-heavy and drop branches or topple over.

Dropped or pruned branches make a wonderful, fragrant hot-burning firewood when seasoned.

Gathering tips: When collecting bay leaves, first look at each branchlet carefully. You want to collect leaves that don't have brown or black spots of honey dew or sooty mold, if possible. Also make sure that the leaves are dense and fresh at the tips and sparser and tougher the closer to the trunk you look. The healthy tougher leaves, farther back on the branch, closer to the trunk, are the ones you want to gather. They will hold their fragrance longer when dried. And the fragrance will hold up much better during cooking, storage, burning, etc.

Use both hands when collecting California bay leaves—one to protect the branch or branchlet from being broken, and the other to carefully pick your leaves. When we take parts of the plants for healing or ritual, it is a good thing to show respect and care for the plant. This energy of respect and care will then carry through to the work at hand.

Cedar

Flat Cedar, Red Cedar, Incense Cedar
(Various botanical names)

Cedar as well as many other conifers are used to consecrate or make Sacred. You can smudge yourself, your space, tools, and clients or patients. The fragrance is both calming and uplifting. Many people connect with their guidance and Spirit Helpers when using this smudge. I prefer incense cedar (*Libocedrus decurrens, Calocedrus decurrens*) because of my special relationship to the plant and its spirit.

The first time I went to the woods to gather smudge without Grandmother, I was hoping to gather cedar and desert sage in a

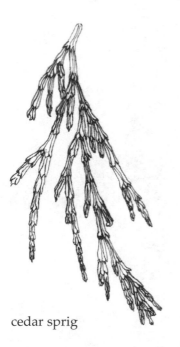

Sacred Way. I wasn't really sure where I wanted to gather. I followed my heart for miles and hours longer than I had intended to drive. When I finally found the right place to stay for the night, it was well past midnight. I promptly crawled into the back of my little blue truck and went to sleep. In the morning I found myself parked under an incense cedar. The sage was growing all around.

I gather cedar both from my special wild places and from places that call to my heart. I always ask and only take a little from each plant, with thankfulness!

cedar sprig

Other uses: Incense cedar is one of the woods sought out as a "hearth board" or "fire block" for fire making. Twirling sticks are variously made from *Artemisia tridentata*, pine, elderberry, and the flower stalk of cattail, among others. Tinder to catch the little coals thus pro-

47

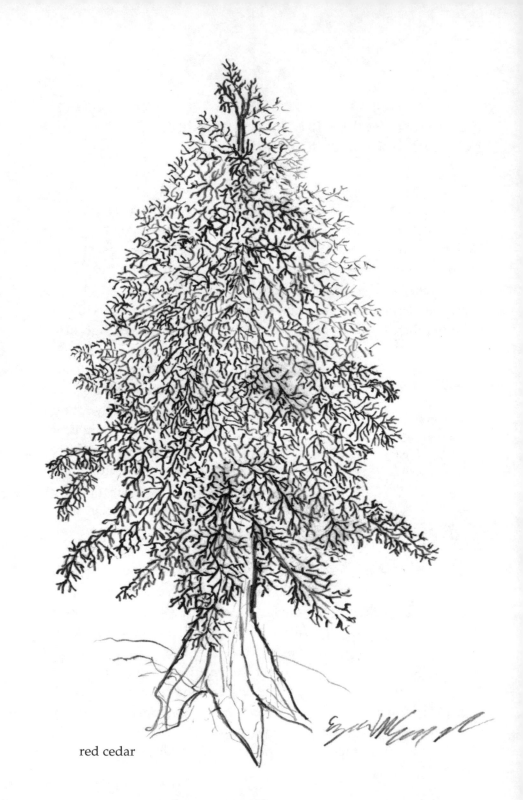

red cedar

duced can be made from cottonwood fluff, cattail fluff, the dried and shredded inner bark of various trees, and the bark of *Artemisia tridentata*.

Commonly a nest is made of shredded bark, which is then lined with the fluff of cattail, cottonwood, or some other similar plant material. When the twirling stick has been used against the hearth board and a small coal has developed, this is tapped loose into the nest and blown on to make it grow. Once you have a little flame it is used to light a prepared nest of tinder and kindling. Now you are well on your way to having a warm fire.

The wood from most cedars can also be split very thin, down to ¼" or less, and used as a basket material, or to make bent wood baskets as was occasionally done in the Klamath area. The wood from red cedar (*Thuja plicata*) was used to make bows for boys here in the Pacific Northwest. Yew wood (*Taxus brevifolia*) was a favored bow wood for men according to some sources.

Cedar leaves and twigs are often used as a medicine associated with the sweat lodge. They are sometimes offered to the fire, brought prepared as smudge or loose in a pouch for the sweat leader, or as an offering for the altar. They are sometimes used in the water that is poured on the rocks in the sweat. The water that is drunk in the sweat lodge may have cedar steeping in it, making a mild cold infusion. Cedar leaves and twigs may be taken into the lodge to wash or scrape the body with, the sweat thus accumulated then flicked into the fire of a dry sweat, or onto the rocks in a plains-style sweat. This kind of doctoring may be done by a healer or sweat leader for an ill individual or, in other instances, an individual may bring their own medicine in to take care of themselves in this way.

Cedar leaves have been used externally for skin conditions and muscle aches. They can be infused in oil or animal fat for this purpose. Incense cedar makes a pleasant tea when infused in hot water. This tea has traditionally been used for colds and flu, and as a pleasing beverage.

Other varieties of cedar include *Thuja occidentalis*, *Chamaecyparis lawsoniana*, and *Thuja plicata*. They are often used in much the same way that California incense cedar is used. I have recently run across references that some of these cedars may be toxic, and especially that they may be unsafe during pregnancy. Some of them may actually have been used as birth control agents in ancient times.

The inner bark of the cedar is used for a large number of purposes. It can be twisted into rope, prepared as a basket material, used to produce mats and rugs, and at one time was used to produce sandals, sacks, and articles of clothing. The inner bark of cedar can be shredded and used as tinder when making fire traditionally. It was once gathered in the spring and prepared as a food.

Cedar wood is also used to make a variety of implements and structures, both utilitarian and Sacred. Traditional houses are constructed from cedar wood, as are boats, floats for fishing nets, and sticks for cooking fish. Cedar wood boxes are still much used to store feathers and smudging supplies. Seasoned cedar wood makes an excellent hot fragrant firewood.

Growing tips: You can grow your own cedar tree if you have good drainage and ample moisture for the young tree until it gets established. When the trees are very young they prefer a little afternoon shade. Once established they are drought-tolerant and can with-stand full sun, hot summers, and snowy winters. Make sure you give your young tree plenty of room to grow up and out. They can reach up to 150 feet in height with a spread of up to 50 feet.

Gathering tips: When collecting cedar, first make sure you have all appropriate permissions. I prefer to use nicely sharpened clippers, because it causes less damage to the tree. Look at the lower branches (on older trees they will be the only ones you can see). Back about 18 inches to 2½ feet you should see some short branchlets about 6-12 inches long with a woody attachment to the main branch. Look closely at the area where your branchlet attaches. You should see a woody structure called a branch bark collar. It looks a little like a turtleneck sweater. When clipping off your branchlet leave that collar behind. It will help protect the tree from infection.

You can usually take one to three branchlets from 3 or 4 branches from a well-established tree. This should not cause the tree any harm. Using your own common sense and intuition is very important.

Juniper

(Juniperus scopulorum, Juniperus occidentalis)

Juniper stands at the top of the world. Her branches caress the Sky with sacred perfume. Her roots embrace the rocky, bare breast of the Earth. She seeks the high, open, bare places, so that she may commune with the elements and the directions without interference.

When we burn juniper smudge we come in contact with a special energy in the universe and in ourselves. We face the elements a little more bravely. Juniper whispers to us about thunderstorms and torrential rains, about gale-force winds and forest fires, about freezing winters at ten thousand feet and the desert's summer swelter. She teaches us to dance with the elements while holding our center, our connection to Earth. She teaches us to survive. She teaches us to stand before Spirit with a bare heart, hiding nothing.

It is this bare heart, this bravery in the face of fear, this willingness to survive, to be part of the dance of life—no matter what the odds, that draws Spirit near.

There are many ways you can invite juniper to help with your inner work: A bundle of juniper hanging by your bed, a small handful of crumbled leaves in a muslin bag slipped in your pillow case, a bit of juniper in a medicine pouch worn as a necklace, a pinch burned as part of your prayers, a sip of fragrant tea as you read.

Other uses: Juniper has been a special medicine plant of the American Indians for thousands of years. The berries from the juniper tree are much used throughout their range as food, beverage, medicine, flavoring, and articles of adornment. The berries were dried and pounded whole, seeds and all, to produce a flour that was used to make a fragrant bread. The berries are still very much in use to brew tea, to help adapt to increases in altitude, as a remedy for urinary and reproductive tract problems, and simply as a refreshing beverage. The twigs and leaves of juniper have been brewed for tea for various ailments, including asthma. The berries

51

are used to flavor meat stews, gravies, and sauces. They are sometimes inserted just under the surface of fish or meat before grilling or cooking to flavor the meat. (Remove before serving—or you might break a tooth!) Whole berries or sometimes, just the woody seed inside, are drilled and made into fragrant beads for jewelry.

The wood of the juniper is often used in construction and for fencing, because of its resistance to rot. Straight boughs from young juniper are used for arrows. Downed juniper is highly valued as a firewood. When seasoned, juniper wood provides for a hot fragrant fire. Juniper is much esteemed as a ceremonial firewood in many areas. When available it is sometimes still used to heat the rocks of sweat lodges as well as for other ceremonial fires.

Juniper's soft bark is employed in fire starting, basketry, diapering babies, and feminine hygiene.

The species of juniper used traditionally include *Juniperus scopulorum* and *Juniperus occidentalis*. Other species may also be used traditionally, but are not mentioned as smudge in the literature. During the training I have been involved with through my grandmother and other traditional people, knowing the exact species of a plant was never stressed. However, certain other knowledge is considered very important. Color, shape, fragrance, texture, and many other types of cues are used to distinguish useful plants from those which may be useless or dangerous. In the absence of a traditional teacher it is best to stick with an exact species identification.

Gathering tips: It is particularly important to obtain all legal permissions to gather juniper, unless you grow your own. Juniper is protected by law in much of its range. It is very slow-growing and very slow to reproduce. Juniper has been nearly eliminated from much of its range by over-harvesting for firewood and other uses.

When gathering juniper I like to use a sharp pair of short-handled garden pruners. Follow the instructions under gathering for cedar to best protect the plants.

Growing tips: Juniper can be grown in a dry sunny spot in the garden or home landscape. It is relatively slow-growing, and is one of those plants that too much kindness will kill. Eventually mature specimens can reach 20-40 feet in height, with about half that spread. In the home garden most of us will likely see our juniper specimens reach between about 8-15 feet. Look up whenever you plant trees. Think tall and don't plant right under the eaves of buildings or too close to power or phone lines.

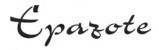

Epazote

(*Chenopodium ambrosioides*)
Also called Mexican Tea and Jerusalem Oak

Epazote helps one to establish healthy boundaries. When as a result of abuse or poor self-esteem, you have pulled in on yourself, or have given up your boundaries entirely, epazote can be helpful.

Its energy is about establishing flowing boundaries that respond to the environment. Try a bundle by your bed or a pinch in your smudge pot. (More is not better when working with epazote, tiny amounts are all that is needed.)

For smudge, harvest before the plants set seeds. The tiny seeds pop and spark when burnt. The leaves are the best part to use for seasoning and tea, while the not yet flowering tops are best to bundle for smudge—or just to hang around and keep you company.

Native to the Yucatan, epazote is believed by many botanists to have established itself in California without human intervention. Given the number of uses for which natives of the Yucatan employ epazote, and the high population of Mexican Americans in California, I am not so sure. I am glad that it chooses to share this environment, so I can accept its Medicine Gift.

Other uses: No matter how you use epazote, a little goes a long way. This herb is used as a seasoning in small amounts. Two or three of its tiny leaves will add subtle flavor to a whole pot of beans and help aid in their digestion. This is one of those nice bean herbs that reduce toot. It can also be used to flavor butter for use with seafood or artichokes. Just remember that a little goes a long way. This is a powerful medicine. Any internal use other than the tiny amounts used for seasoning should be occasional and sparing.

Traditionally epazote tea was used to expel worms, and for coughs, congestion, and inflammation. Using the essential oil for treatment of worms is dangerous. It has been reported that as few as four drops of the essential oil can kill a young child if taken internally.

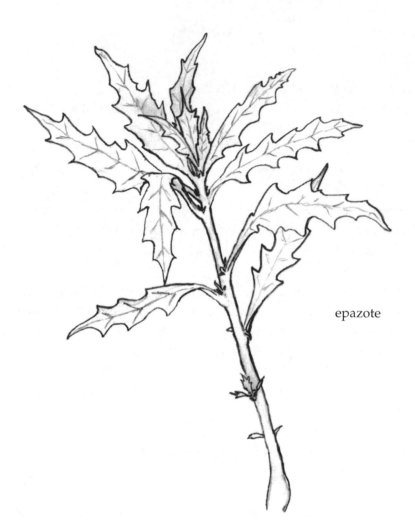

epazote

Growing tips: Epazote is not a plant most people would grow for its good looks. It rather resembles a weed. Epazote reaches about 18 inches tall and spreads out about the same distance in several directions. However, if given plenty of water, it will likely grow larger and be less fragrant. The flowers are very tiny and green. Unless you understand a bit about botany or plant growth and look close, you probably wouldn't think it flowers at all.

Epazote is a tender perennial. It dies back to its roots in the winter in temperate zones, and is grown as an annual in cold northern or mountainous regions. Epazote likes full sun. It can be grown in a variety of soils. I have found it growing in the wild in sand and in hard-pan. It is not too particular about soil. Give it ample water and good drainage when young. Once established it will thrive on benign neglect.

If the tiny but copious flowers are allowed to set seed, you may well have a thousand new epazote plants come spring. For those who don't have a thousand friends in need of epazote, you can clip back your plants before they set seed or make use of a hoe early in the spring. Epazote sends down deep roots. Unwanted but well-established plants can be hard to remove.

Epazote is a little difficult to identify in the wild, as there are many other weedy species it resembles. Unless you have a knowledgeable person to help you identify this plant, I recommend growing your own epazote, or checking out well-stocked herb shops or Mexican grocery stores.

Fennel

(*Foeniculum vulgare*)

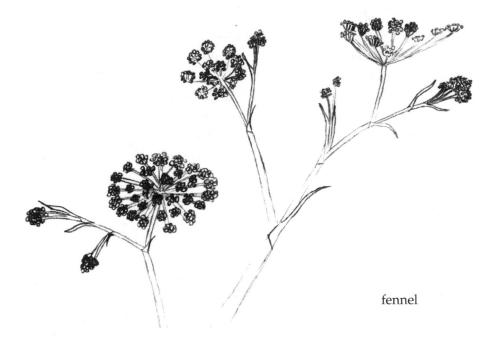

fennel

Fennel flowers, seeds, stalks, or leaves are equally effective used as smudge. Fennel can be gathered from the wild, purchased, or grown in the home garden. Europeans have used fennel for food, medicine, and to repel evil energies since the Middle Ages. It can be incorporated with other herbs to burn as smudge, hung over the door or near the bed, or carried in a small medicine pouch.

Be aware that it looks similar to poison hemlock, and the two are often found growing side by side. Poison hemlock's scent varies from a bland green smell to the distinctive scent of a mouse nest. Its stems are often marked with red and its flowers are white to greenish to cream in color. Fennel smells strongly of licorice, its stems are solid green, and its flowers are bright yellow. However, almost every year someone poisons themselves with poison hemlock after collecting "fennel." Make sure the plants you gather from are truly fennel and that they are not inter-growing with poison hemlock.

Fennel is found near rivers and streams, vacant lots, and along roadways. Leaves or flowers can be snipped or snapped off and incorporated with other herbs in smudge sticks. Seeds can be massaged or rubbed off their stems and burned on commercially prepared charcoal or thrown onto the embers of a fire.

Other uses: Fennel is well known as a digestive aid, and as such it is used as a tea and a flavoring for food. Fresh or dry leaves or the seeds can be used to make tea or employed as a seasoning. Fennel tea is often given to colicky babies as a gentle remedy. When my son was young I would give him the fibrous stalks to use for teething. The fennel helped numb his gums and calm his mood. I always held him on my lap and kept a close eye, in case he chewed a piece loose that he might choke on.

Fennel tea is a gentle remedy for female problems. Some people find it helpful for PMS, the postpartum blues, cramps, and absent or scanty periods. Fennel tea is one of those remedies that can be helpful for people with irregular and troublesome moon times.

Fennel makes a lovely addition to a wild flower border or the back of a large flower bed. It can reach five feet tall or more, and has fragrant fern-like foliage and lacy yellow flowers. These flowers make a wonderful flavorful tea or an interesting addition to a salad. Once established, fennel will tolerate or even thrive with neglect. Fennel flowers attract bees and butterflies. Fennel honey is a delight for anyone who loves sweet licorice. Some of the butterflies attracted will stay to lay their eggs among fennel's abundant greenery. If you find caterpillars crawling around and eating some of your fennel, I do hope you will share. They are next year's beautiful butterflies.

Fennel seed can be purchased at many healthfood and herb shops. If not available in your area, you can order plants or seeds and grow your own.

Mint

(*Mentha, Monarda,* various species)

The mints are both cleansing and uplifting. They can be burned either alone or incorporated with other herbs. My preference is to add a small amount of mint to my basic cedar and sage mixture. I use either a sprig or two of wild mint or prunings from those grown in my yard. (See "Words of Caution.")

Other uses: The mints and monardas are a very variable, closely related group of plants. They have traditionally been used in the treatment of ailments, as pleasant beverages, and to season food. Many mints and monardas have been traditionally made into tea to drink and also used as compresses for colds, inflammation, and headache.

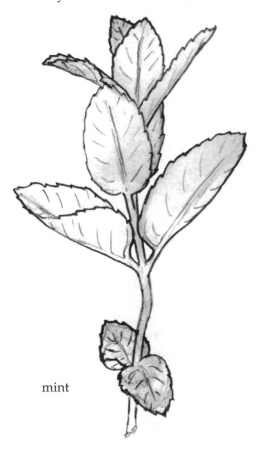

mint

Some of the traditional medicinal uses of the tea include treatments for indigestion, heartburn, stomachache, nausea, colds and flu, headache, and migraine. If you plan on using the mints or monardas internally, please be sure of the botanical name of the specific plant you plan to use. Then do a little research on the uses and safety of the specific plant you plan to use. Some mints, especially the pennyroyals, are known to cause miscarriage.

Mints and monardas have also been used as components

of salves and ointments as well as pounded and used for poultices and facials.

I use mint in herb tea blends for colds and flu, stomach upset, flatulence, headache, and simply because we enjoy the taste. Many people find it helpful for heartburn, but I find it often makes that problem worse. The essential oils naturally present in the plant relax the sphincter muscles. This can cause gastric juices to escape the stomach into the esophagus and cause that awful burning sensation. Not everyone has this reaction to mint tea. I find it only to be a problem if I already have heartburn. But I think it is good information to keep in the back of your mind.

Growing mints: Most mints and monardas prefer moist soils and partial shade. Monardas like a little humus in a soil that is not too heavy and most will tolerate quite a bit of sun. Most of the mints will grow in anything from clay to sand as long as it is moist. They are famous for their ability to spread by runners and by reseeding. And they are difficult to control. Think about this before planting them in your garden.

I enjoy mints planted along the edge of the lawn. I allow them to spread as they will and simply mow whatever grows into the mower's path. If you enjoy a tidier landscape, carefully read your plant catalogs or ask thoughtful questions at your local nursery. Not all varieties are invasive and some may be more suited to your climate than others.

Gathering mints: As with all other plants, make sure you are gathering somewhere it is legal to do so, and that you have all necessary permissions. Be aware of what occupies higher ground from your gathering spot. Will water flow or seep from roads, chemically treated agricultural areas, or from some other source of chemical or natural pollution? These thoughts are good to keep in mind whenever you gather materials.

I like to use a sharp knife or pair of clippers when gathering for smudge. I cut or clip the plant to about the length I will use in my bundles. I like to use the flowering tops while they are still colorful and before they set seed. The seeds from the mints, as well as from most of the plants used for smudge, will pop and spark if burned. This is not such a great thing for your clothing or furnishings!

Some of the hybrid varieties of the monardas have flowers that are too large to be used in this way. From these plants you can choose non-flowering sprigs.

When gathering from my own plants for tea or other medicinal preparations, I simply pinch the top below the first or second set of leaves. I use mints fresh by pouring boiling water over them and steeping for about 10 minutes.

Our winters are usually mild enough that I can find a few fresh leaves all winter long. If you have deep snow you may want to gather some mint to dry for winter use.

Mugwort

(*Artemisia vulgaris*)
Wormwood, River Sage, Cronewort

Mugwort is a California native, with similar species found in many parts of the world. It is used for healing, divination, and to stimulate dreams and visions nearly everywhere it occurs. If you have ever had moxibustion during acupuncture or other healing work, the herbs burned are most likely the Japanese or Chinese species of mugwort.

In the California Indian community this plant is most often called wormwood. In central California it is often the preferred herb to burn and use as offerings before and during sweats. It is bundled and used as smudge for many ceremonies. It is often the herb infused in the sweat house water offered to the rocks and for the participants to drink and pour over their heads. Mugwort is also used as a poultice for bruises, sprains, poison oak, and infections.

Mugwort is important to European healers. I was once showing a friend my plants and herbs when she asked, "Do you have mugwort growing here by your door?"

"Yes, a little bit, but I keep pulling it out, I have more over here beneath my bedroom window."

"Oh, you shouldn't pull it out! It wants to be here. In European tradition, it is called cronewort, and they say it likes to grow at the doors of healers."

Mugwort bundles can be hung by your bed, or burned before sleep or during ritual. Some people find the smoke to be slightly mind-altering. As with any potentially mind-altering substance, avoid its use if you plan on driving, operating machinery, or have an infant or other dependent person in your care, until you are certain how you will react. I gather my mugwort, with care and respect, from wild plants, or from the special ones beneath my window when they need to be trimmed. Mugwort is UNSAFE FOR PREGNANCY.

Growing tips: Mugwort tolerates many soil types, but it needs to have ample soil moisture during winter through spring. Once established it will tolerate summer drought and simply die back to the roots after flowering.

Plants reach from 3-5 feet in height, and will die back to the ground after producing an abundance of tiny green flowers. They are best grown at the back of the garden because of their height, or alone along a fence or wall. The plants will slowly spread by underground stems. When your stand gets too thick or large, plants can be divided and shared with friends.

Other uses: The leaves reportedly can be used in cooking and are considered a bitter digestive herb. Mugwort is closely related to tarragon, but has a flavor more reminiscent of oregano. Long ago when I was a mere kid in my early 20s, and before I was clean and sober, I used to fix a huge batch of spaghetti well seasoned with mugwort about once a month. All my buddies enjoyed that spaghetti, and for those of us who were sensitive to the mild mind-altering properties, it was a bit like having a couple of glasses of wine. That was a long time ago.

I do not recommend using mugwort in food. It is considered UNSAFE FOR PREGNANCY. As a now, long-time clean and sober person, I, for one, would resent being served food with possible mind-altering ingredients.

Mugwort is an effective mosquito repellent. When hiking you can rub fresh mugwort leaves on all exposed skin and then carry the bruised leaves in your pocket. The treatment tends to need repeating every ½ hour or so. (This is most effective if at least one member of your group does not use the mugwort. Hungry skeeters are going to bite someone. If you stink to their way of smelling and someone else smells yummy—well—you know who is going to get bit!)

Mugwort is also my very favorite poison oak remedy. I have seen fresh ground-up mugwort poultice work miracles on very bad cases of poison oak. It is most effective if you can gather the mugwort from near where the person got into the poison oak. This really seems to work the best, but it is not always possible. Mugwort can also be

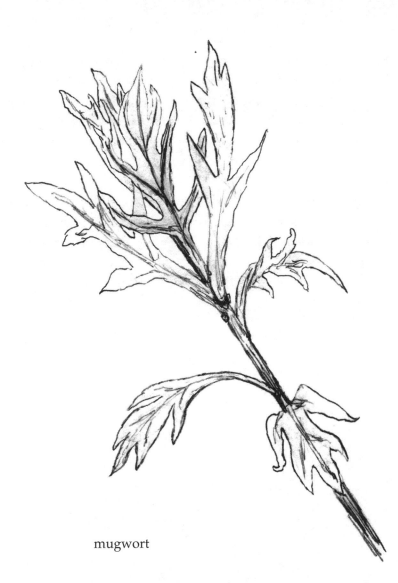

mugwort

extracted in apple cider vinegar and used as a lotion on poison oak. This is nearly as effective as fresh mugwort and can be prepared ahead, as it has a long shelf life.

In many years of working with herbs, I have run across one person who was allergic to mugwort, and one case of poison oak that did not respond to mugwort. Pay attention whenever trying natural remedies. Be ready to try a different remedy or seek professional advice if you don't see noticeable improvement.

Gathering tips: I like to use a sharp pair of garden pruners and clip the stalk the exact length needed for a smudge bundle or for whatever purpose I have in mind. Smudge is best made before the plant produces seeds, as they sometimes spark when burned, and some people are allergic to the fuzz that helps the seeds drift on the breeze. If I am making a poultice I remove the top few inches if tender or simply a few juicy leaves from each stem.

Mugwort cut after the end of the rainy season and before flowering will probably not regenerate and set seed, unless it is rooted near a source of water. Keep this in mind when collecting. Grandmother always reminded me that every plant has the right to reproduce. Only cut a few stems from each stand of wild mugwort, and make a mental note of where to collect a root to start your own next winter.

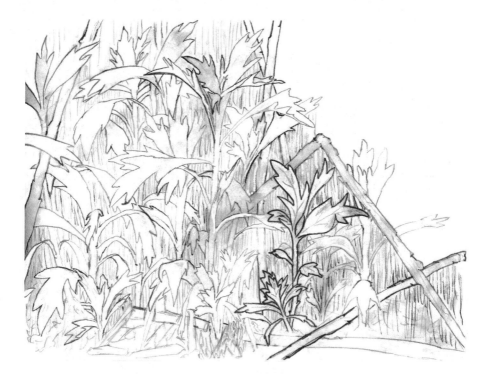

Mugwort community with spring growth in last year's stems.

Mullein

(*Verbascum thapsus*)
Velvet Plant, Torchweed

Mullein grows wild over much of the industrialized world. Its special spiritual work is to heal the damage created by human activity. It is not uncommon to see a large plant growing where a recent road cut fords a stream. The mullein stands ready to cast its seeds upon any subsequent erosion. The roots help to hold the soil in place, and the furry leaves attract and hold dust and wind-blown soil. Mice and insects find shelter, food, and protection under the spreading leaves of the mullein plant. Not only are the leaves eaten by many creatures, but the nectar from the flowers and the copious supply of seeds provide for many. Life encourages life. The waste products of the mice and insects enrich and rebuild the soil. Given time, mullein and her helpers will heal the damaged land.

The work mullein has to do in the wild is very important. I am careful not to interfere out of selfishness or self-centeredness. When I collect mullein from the wild I take only a single leaf from each plant, after seeking each plant's permission.

I bundle my leaves together, often using four leaves, one for each direction.

I burn a pinch or two at a time—either on charcoal, or by holding a leaf so that a small surface rests in a candle flame. I inhale the smoke, and direct it to my heart or the area of myself or my patient that needs healing. I use it for healing trauma that originates out of relationships with other people, or for protection in new endeavors. Most people find the smoke to be very grounding and calming. (See "Words of Caution.")

Other uses: Mullein leaves are a well-known remedy for coughs and bronchitis. Tea made from the leaves is very soothing in cases where the coughing has become painful. Mullein-infused oil also makes a nice base for a soothing chest rub for muscles that have become sore from coughing. For very young children or for those feeling very sick, you might try barely simmering a large pot of strong mullein tea at the back of your stove. I have found that this often helps relieve painful coughs.

Mullein flowers are infused in olive oil as a remedy for earache. I know lots of people who swear by this remedy. Tea from the roots is a traditional remedy for urinary infections. (If you have chronic or recurring infections, those that do not respond to natural remedies within two days, cause noticeable pain, or if the patient is a child, please seek professional attention.)

The flowering stalks, before setting seed, are brewed into a tea for soothing frazzled nerves. This is a stay-at-home remedy. All parts of the mullein plant can cause drowsiness, but the flowering tops produce the strongest effect.

Mullein is used as a dye plant producing yellow, bronze, and gray dyes. The dried stalks have been employed in fire starting, and they are sometimes dipped in tallow or pitch to form a ceremonial torch.

Growing tips: Mullein is not too particular about the soil type it grows in. Like other weedy plants it prefers disturbed soil, so the edges of a garden are a likely spot for mullein to thrive. If you garden on a slight slope, so much the better. Mullein likes the moisture from a nearby garden, but also does the best when good drainage is allowed for.

Mullein is a biannual. Generally it takes 2 years for a plant to produce seed. The first year mullein produces a rosette of soft gray green leaves (sometimes referred to as "backpackers' TP.") In rich soil with ample water and good drainage a single plant may form a clump up to 3 feet across or more.

The second year a flower stalk grows from the center of the leaves and the leaves begin to wither. The flower stalk may reach from 3-6 feet in height and open a few bright yellow flowers a day for the entire summer season. These flowers are attractive to butterflies and hummingbirds, and will produce a copious supply of seeds. After the stalk is completely dry you can shake out the seeds wherever you want to invite mullein to grow. The following spring, after flowering, a few small plants may sprout from the base of the old mullein stalk. More often though, the original plant dies.

Gathering tips: Make sure you have all appropriate permissions before gathering. You also want to chose a site that is free of chemical contamination. When gathering from wild plants I only collect one leaf from each plant. I firmly hold the leaf near its base and if the plant does not seem to object I gently twist it from the stem. If collecting from a young plant that is still a basal rosette, I take hold of the leaf stem and pull straight up. Flowering stalks can be gathered, if you have a large stand, by clipping with sharp garden pruners. Roots are best dug as flowering begins, from your own garden, if you have several plants. After the roots are washed the whole plant can be hung upside down to dry, after removing some of the leaves for smudge bundles.

Pine, Fir, Hemlock

(Various botanical names)

These conifers are burnt for their purifying and cleansing effect. Many people use pine, especially piñon pine, alone. I sometimes incorporate pine, fir, hemlock, or spruce with the other herbs I'm using for smudge.

I often gather a shoot or two from the trees growing near where I am collecting herbs, or use the prunings from trees growing in my yard.

Pine

Other uses: Certain pine trees produce edible nuts, such as the sugar pine and piñon pine. However, many of these trees and their seeds are now protected. Unless you have treaty rights to collect them you will have to grow them. This is a long, slow process.

The Italian stone pine is a faster-growing species that has been brought into cultivation. In Italy and other places, pine nuts are produced commercially as an export crop and are available in specialty markets in many parts of the world.

In times of acorn shortage or corn crop failure the mucilaginous parts of the inner bark of various trees are utilized for food. The ponderosa pine is one favored tree for this in the California region. It can be cooked into soup, or dried and used to prepare flour for bread. At times other than emergency the inner bark of certain trees is used to make tea or gruel for people who are invalid, malnourished, or recovering from illness.

Pine needles, particularly from those species of pine with long needles, are used for weaving baskets. Traditionally these baskets are used for storing seeds and grain, as well as other items that may be attractive to insects. The naturally occurring essential oils released

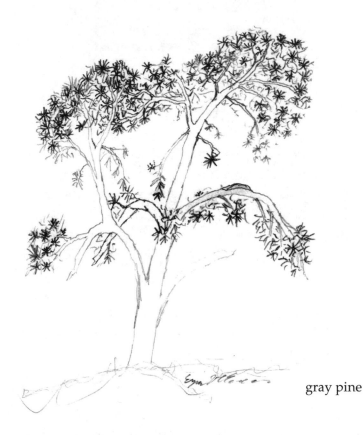

gray pine

over time by the dried pine needles are an effective deterrent for most insect pests. Depending on the basket traditions of individual tribes, pine needle baskets may be coiled or twinned, the latter being more difficult. The coiled baskets may consist of open work, which allows the pine needles to show as a design element, or they may be completely covered by other intricate design materials. Pine needle baskets of various types are still produced and often made available for purchase.

In some areas pine needle baskets are covered with pitch, dried, and used to store water. A friend of mine grew up drinking water from a pitched basket. She maintains that the water from those baskets was the best water she has ever tasted.

The wood from various pines was and is used for utilitarian pur-

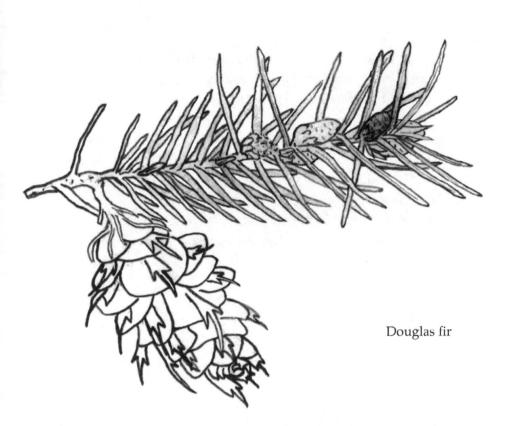

Douglas fir

poses by many tribes. These uses include boat making, fire starting, home construction, producing implements such as spoons, etc. A knobby branch was sometimes employed in making a torch. Various species were used in this way, especially *Pinus contorta* if available, because of the high pitch level of its wood. The inner bark of various species as well as the roots are employed in basket making. A few species of pine were tapped in the spring. The sweet saps obtained were primarily used medicinally rather than as a sweetener. However, sugar was occasionally prepared from the sap.

Some tribes use pine nuts for ornamentation, producing beautiful jewelry and regalia. Indian and natural history museums often have jewelry and other articles on display and for sale that incorporate carefully prepared pine nuts with other natural materials.

Fir

The inner bark of the fir tree was used to dye hides. It produced a color similar to our modern tan-colored leather. A very pleasant tea can be brewed from its leaves. I enjoy fir leaf tea whenever I go camping.

The tea is sometimes used in the sweat lodge, both to drink and sprinkled on the rocks. Sometimes twigs with leaves will be taken into the sweat lodge to wash or scrape off sweat. Fir used in this way is considered a medicine for muscle and joint pain.

The tea, particularly from Douglas fir, was once employed against venereal disease. (Today I would advise seeing a doctor, and taking the proper precautions so that you can avoid needing a cure in the first place.)

Hemlock

The bark of hemlock trees, particularly *Tsuga heterophylla*, can be used for tanning hides, and the inner bark of this tree also served as a survival food.

Growing tips: Evergreen trees tend to thrive in the home landscape and are readily available from most nurseries. Good drainage is helpful. Use ample summertime irrigation until the young pine trees are well established. Long, slow, deep watering on an infrequent basis will help develop a deep root system and a more stable adult tree. Keep an eye on your young trees. Don't let them become water stressed as it will make them more susceptible to disease.

Look up before you plant. Most evergreen trees will eventually get quite tall. Make sure you are not planting them beneath an overhanging balcony or power lines. Also think about what is underneath the ground. Avoid planting them over your leach line or septic system, over underground cables, or directly over your plumbing or drainage system.

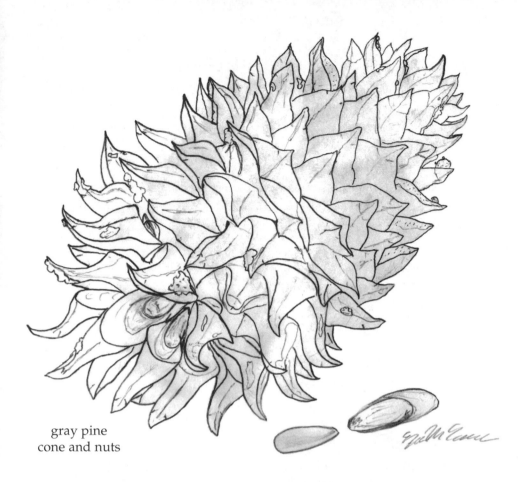

gray pine
cone and nuts

Gathering tips: After making sure you have all appropriate permissions, look at your tree carefully. Take hold of a single branch and look for branchlets growing back close to the trunk. You want a healthy looking branchlet, but not one of the dominant growers. Choose one that is about the length you need for your intended purpose. A sharp pair of garden clippers is a must, unless you are going to collect needles a few at a time. Next examine the area where the branchlet connects to the main branch. You are looking for something called the branch bark collar. It looks a bit like a bark turtleneck sweater right near where the branchlet connects to the branch. You want to leave that structure intact when you clip your branchlet off. It serves an immune function for the tree. However, you want to only leave about ½ inch of branch protruding from the collar, so you don't leave a large area to foster the growth of insects or fungi.

If you are collecting needles for baskets or potpourri, the best ones are already dry but still hanging on the tree. Use your hands to gently loosen them. It will take a little practice, but eventually you will find that you can easily remove them without harm to the tree.

Resin, Balsam, Gum, Sap

(Various origins)

I gather dried droplets of resin from various forest trees to use for smudge and healing. I never collect the sap that is closing a wound, and I try to avoid any that is still gooey. I am partial to resins from pine, juniper, fir, and spruce trees. People also use sweet gum, birch, and acacia, among others. Some examples of commercially available resins are benzoin, copal, dragon's blood, frankincense, and myrrh.

Resins embody the four elements when used as smudge or incense. Water is pulled from the Earth by the tree's roots and transformed into sap. The tree grows from Mother Earth to Father Sky, offering its fragrance to the realms of both Sky and Earth. The sap as resin embodies the elements of Earth and Water and their movement towards the Sky.

When burning we introduce the element of Fire, and as the resin transforms into smoke, it becomes Air. Symbolically and actually, we are affirming and partaking of our connection to all creation when we prayerfully inhale the Sacred Smoke of our chosen resin.

Other uses: Traditionally certain resins are associated with particular ailments, or used most frequently in particular contexts. While much of this information is lost, a little remains. Pine resin, particularly that of the sugar pine, was burned for the treatment of coughs, colds, and rheumatism. The smoke is used to wash the body, from head to toe.

Pitch from various trees was traditionally cooked with animal fat to produce a salve for infections and inflammation. My grandmother was not too particular as to what conifer her pitch came from. Gathering it was more a prayerful process and not associated with a particular species. She usually prepared her poultices with coconut oil, but always talked about how traditionally we would have used animal fat.

Grandmother followed one of the branches of the Ghost Dance religion. She believed that one day all the colonists and all their things would disappear. It was important to her that I know how things should be done.

I now clarify animal fat by boiling in mild vinegar water baths and allowing it to harden in between. I scrape the impurities from the top and bottom of the the fat and use clean water with a bit of vinegar and reboil repeatedly until the fat comes out clean. I pressure-can this in small jars to use for making salve.

Resins and sap from trees were also employed for more mundane things, like glue. There is evidence that various firs, including *Abies mertensiana*, were used in this way.

Pine resin, as well as other resins, has been used as a glue in utilitarian objects, in artwork such as turquoise mosaics, and as a glaze for pottery as well as for waterproofing.

Resins, particularly those from pine, have been used as a "chewing gum." I have had elders direct me to chew "pine gum" for mouth sores, sinus infections, sore throats, earaches, etc. If you want to try this, make sure the pine you choose is free of pesticides and other toxins, and that it is considered an edible species. (Sugar pine, gray or bull pine, ponderosa pine, and Jeffrey pine are pretty safe bets. However, there is never any accounting for individual reactions or personal allergies.)

The resin from balsam fir or *Abies lasiocarpa* was used as an application to soften corns and calluses and made into a tea for lung problems.

Growing tips: See section on "Pine, Fir, Hemlock."

Gathering tips: The first tip I am going to give you is, don't get the pitch on your clothes! You are going to do it anyway, even though I told you not to, so wear old clothes and don't wash them with clothes you care about. With a little practice you can almost always tell which drops of resin are dry and which are still sticky. Baby oil and rubbing alcohol are about the best for removing sap and pitch from your hands and hair.

Besides picking the tiny globs off tree bark, if you burn firewood you may have another source. Sometimes some of the wood has thick seams of pitch running through it. A clean putty knife or butter knife can be employed to remove this pitch. It can be cut into small pieces to dry in a protected place, or stored in an airtight container almost indefinitely.

Please treat any pitch or resin you are storing very carefully. These materials are extremely flammable.

Root

Root is a mysterious plant substance used primarily in private tribe-specific ceremonies. In recent years it has begun to appear at powwows and other public events. Root is burned and sometimes carried in pouches or chewed for healing, cleansing, protecting, and blessing. Specific uses vary from tribe to tribe.

The mysterious thing about root is that it is gathered and prepared only by very specific individuals within a tribe's tradition. For some tribes this person may receive the distinction through heredity and in others the job may be assigned by a specific elder.

These plants are not identified by species. In fact, not all members of a specific species would be considered "root." In many traditions only material gathered and prepared from a specific stand by the appropriate individual is "root."

This is not a do-it-yourself medicine. I have included it here only because it is something you might be exposed to at a powwow, sweat, or other event.

Other uses: According to ethnographic data, some root may be osha—*Ligusticum porteri*. Osha is also chewed or brewed into tea for colds, flu, and other ailments where stimulating the immune system is helpful. A poultice of the tea, mashed root, or greens is used for muscle and joint pain and injuries. Another plant that may be "root" for some people is *Lomatium dissectum*, or lomation. It is used much the same as the preceding plant.

Growing tips: Plant the seeds in flats of sterilized soil in late fall after the weather has turned cool. Place the flats on an outdoor table or bench and cover with a screen to protect from birds, slugs, and rodents. This screen should let in light and soften the effects of rain, but not entirely protect the seeds from the elements.

These seeds require a long germination period. The alternating cycles of rain and cold, light and dark will stimulate that germination process. Once you have tiny seedlings transplant them to their own containers. When they seem ready to withstand attack by hungry critters plant them out in a bright, well-drained spot.

Keep an eye on your young plants through at least their first spring and early summer. Infrequent deep watering may be necessary if they begin to wilt. After they have flowered and begun to set seed, withhold water. This may take two years.

Your plants will die back to the ground in late summer or fall. When they are dormant, avoid giving them supplementary water. You should have new sprouts in the spring for a few years. By then, if they are happy, you should begin to get some volunteer seedlings from seeds set the year before.

Gathering tips: These plants should not be gathered from the wild. They are easily mistaken for a number of poisonous plants. They are also protected throughout much of their range. These considerations are in addition to the cultural considerations already mentioned.

Once you have an established bed you can dig your own roots in spring or fall. This will be easiest on the bed if done while the plants are dormant—either after they have gone to sleep in the fall or before they wake up in the spring.

Thoroughly clean your roots and then slice and dry completely to prevent spoilage. Store them in airtight containers until needed.

You can grow your own osha or lomation, or purchase commercially prepared root, but it would be inappropriate to represent what you grow or purchase as "root" in the context of traditional ceremony or healing.

Sage, Desert

(*Artemisia tridentata*)

This plant is called sage brush, black sage (for its seeds), and white sage (for its appearance). It is used interchangeably with various other artemisias and salvias for their ability to clear both negative and foreign energy and entities from oneself, one's environment, or one's tools.

My first affirmation came with a gift of a dried and pressed sprig of sage. Every time I smelled that sprig, and indeed every time I smell desert sage, I am reminded that "I am all right, right now!" (Remember, all there is, is now!) As with all the herbs I gather, I proceed in a Sacred Way with respect and thankfulness.

Other uses: Wood from various sages (both artemisias and salvias) are used to produce flutes, whistles, prayer sticks, prayer arrows, and other religious objects.

For headache, sage tea and sage poultices are used on the temples and forehead. If you have lots of sage, several cups of strong tea can be placed in your bath water. Sometimes burning a sage leaf or two, or rubbing a little diluted essential oil on your temples and at the back of the head will help.

Traditionally a poultice of sage is considered anti-inflammatory and healing. *Artemisia tridentata* was also used as a tea for diarrhea and for colds. I haven't tried it for diarrhea, so I can't speak to how effective it might be. However, I find an occasional cup of sage tea to be invigorating and refreshing and I do find that it is helpful with the symptoms a cold can bring.

Blue and silver sage (*Artemisia cana*) was used as a general tonic, to restore the hair, as a poultice for skin conditions, and the leaves were sometimes chewed to relieve thirst until water could be obtained.

The wood from *Artemisia tridentata* makes a satisfactory fire and cooking wood. In the old days the small strong straight sticks and the crumbled bark were employed in fire making. The bark can be variously prepared to form ropes, baskets, and simple articles of clothing. The shrubs themselves were once piled up and woven together with sage bark rope to provide temporary shelter in hunting and gathering areas.

Growing tips: The desert artemisias all prefer an arid, well-drained environment. However, they do sometimes adapt to life in a neglected landscape. Even here in the temperate rainforest of northern California where we get an average rainfall of about 70 inches a year, they can be grown.

In a moist environment, the lee side of a building away from the onslaught of prevailing winds will provide some protection from excess rain. Plants should be planted where they will get full sun for most of the day. A relatively high spot, where the ground gently slopes away, will help keep their roots dry and prevent rot. If planted near a building, make sure the rain gutters are in good working order to help prevent your plants from getting soaked.

Young sage plants are best planted out in the spring in temperate environments and in the fall in arid desert environments. This will help reduce shock and give your plants the best opportunity to make it through their first year. Once established they should live long lives if they are not over-watered or fertilized.

Gathering tips: My favorite time to gather desert sage is after they have formed their tiny copious flower buds, but just before those buds are fully opened. They are at their most fragrant at this time. In many environments and during most years the sage will reach this stage from mid to late July. Keep an eye on the wild patches you tend or the plants behind your barn.

If gathered too early, before their essence has fully developed, their fragrance will dissipate soon after drying. At this time their moisture content is also high, which prolongs the drying process.

If gathered after the flowers open, they will be laden with pollen, which may cause allergies for some people. And if you should wait until after the sage plants set seed you will find that those tiny seeds which are barely visible will spark and sputter and pop. These little sparks can leave small burn holes in clothing and they are very hot. Watch your plants so you can catch the moment just right.

Sage sprigs of the exact length you wish to use can be snapped or clipped off the bush. If you are gathering from wild plants do so in such a way that the next person along your path will not be able to tell you have been there. Take just a few sprigs from each plant, only with the plant's permission.

Sweet Grass

(*Glyceria fluitans, Glyceria aquatica, Hierochloe odorata*)

This wild grass is found growing on the plains of North America and Russia. The long, delightfully fragrant blades are gathered before frost and braided to form a short rope or long wand. The smoke is commonly used for grounding, protecting, and making Sacred. It is used alone or sometimes in combination with cedar and sage.

Other uses: Sweet grass can be brewed into a fragrant tasty tea which is sometimes used to calm the nerves, settle the stomach, or soothe a sore throat. It is also kept with regalia and ceremonial items to repel insects and ensure the items keep a clean fresh scent.

Sweet grass is also a favored basket material in many cultures. The larger baskets resemble those made of pine needles and the smaller ones resemble those made of horsehair. They exude that delightful sweet grass fragrance.

Sweet grass candles can be made by snipping the braids or left-over bits into tiny pieces and mixing with the melted wax before pouring into the molds, or sprinkled in between sheets of beeswax before rolling around the wick.

The tiny snips of sweet grass are also sometimes added to soap-making ingredients before pouring into molds. Freshly cut sweet grass can be wound around a taper candle or other form and allowed to dry to form curls that can be added to potpourri. These ideas will give you additional ways to make use of sweet grass in a professional office environment.

Growing tips: Sweet grass favors moist yet well-drained sandy soils. Heavy clay soils or those that are very high in organic matter will produce spindly unhappy plants. It can be grown in containers, and depending on your soil, this may be the best method for you. Sweet grass thrives in filtered bright light and will tolerate full sun for part of the day or in northern environments.

Gathering tips: Sweet grass is typically cut when the leaves are mature but before they have begun to yellow. Keep an eye on your plants or the wild patches you tend. Depending on your climate this stage of the plant's life will be reached anywhere from mid-summer to late fall. Plants should be clipped about three inches above the ground. If they are clipped too close to the ground the crown will be damaged and they will not grow back next year. The leaves can be wilted briefly and then braided. Short pieces of sweet grass can be used to tie each end of the braid, so that it won't unravel.

Uva Ursi

(*Arctostaphylos uva-ursi*)
Bearberry

The fragrance and energy of this herb is very calming and grounding. Uva ursi is one of the herbs commonly mixed with tobacco and called kinnikinnik. Another herb often used in kinnikinnik is the red twig dogwood or *Cornus sericea*. This blend is often used for smoking during Pipe Ceremony. This herb is not used to form smudge bundles.

Other uses: Uva ursi tea was traditionally used as a remedy for urinary tract infections and female problems. This tea is useful for excessive menstruation, cramps, menopause, and after childbirth. It is also employed for conditions where there is excess moisture, such as coughs and swellings. The tea makes a pleasant morning beverage and provides an opportunity for variety when alternated with other herbal teas.

Growing tips: Uva ursi is a low growing perennial shrub, often planted as a ground cover. It will grow in full sun or filtered light and it tolerates acid soils. It is considered fire-retardant and drought-tolerant. Plants are readily available at many nurseries and a number of cultivated varieties exist. If planted near an area that gets summer irrigation good drainage is a must, otherwise it is not too fussy about soil or care. Uva ursi is a close but diminutive relative of the manzanita bush and the madrone tree.

Gathering tips: A good sharp pair of garden clippers is a must, unless you are going to gather the tiny leaves one at a time. Positive identification and attention to detail are also important. Uva ursi is often found inter-growing with alpine azaleas and other subshrubs and ground covers. It is a bit difficult to identify, except when it is blooming, which is the wrong time to collect. You might consider growing this one yourself.

Late summer or early fall are my favorite times to gather uva ursi. Leaves should still be bright green and leathery. I study the plants and clip back those portions that will most benefit by the branching that will occur the next year, or thin with the idea of allowing more sun to reach new growth.

Uva ursi sprigs should be dried inside or in the shade. Leaves can then be removed or stored for use.

Wild Tobacco

(*Nicotiana*, various species)

When Grandmother Spider grew lonely for her children, She was born as Thought Woman from a dewdrop resting on a tobacco leaf. Ever since, tobacco has been used to connect with Sacred Beings and Wisdom.

Unprocessed tobacco is smoked, used for smudge, put in medicine bags, and kept with spiritual tools. We often employ it whenever Sacred energy is needed.

In the old days, spitting or blowing doctors sometimes employed decoctions made of tobacco. The fluid was drawn into the mouth of the doctor and spit or blown onto the patient. These kinds of treatments are part of larger ceremonies and regimes for treating various ailments. However, the blowing of tobacco smoke drawn into the mouth from a pipe or rubbing tobacco tea on by hand is much more common than the spitting or blowing of tea.

The first time I had an Indian doctor spit a mouthful of something on me, I was quite shocked, but managed to maintain my composure. It was later explained to me that the fluid, coming from the mouth of the doctor who had been praying and singing for me, was a special blessing. And that knowledge is why I am sharing this with you—so you will know what is going on, if it ever happens to you.

I know of people who have self-treated Lyme disease, spirochetosis, and scabies with tobacco tea. I believe this is a dangerous practice that no one should undertake on their own.

I do not recommend that anyone experiment with putting tobacco tea in their mouth or on their body. Tobacco is a powerful medicine full of potentially dangerous natural chemicals. It needs to be used traditionally and with respect. Traditional doctors have abilities and powers beyond western science. This is a medicine that is not for the rest of us to play around with.

Other uses: Tobacco tea is used to spray on plants for the purpose of killing aphids and other pests. It should be used as a last resort. I am told that the toxins in the tobacco persist and build up in the soil with repeated use, and that those toxins can be absorbed by our garden plants and then be ingested by us.

Some Native people use species of lobelia as tobacco, or in much the same way as tobacco. This herb should also be used with caution, however, small amounts are occasionally used internally to lower a fever.

Growing tips: There are actually many types of wild tobacco. Most of them are relatively easy to grow. I find that it thrives in ordinary flower beds and will set copious seed and take over if you turn your back too long. Wild tobacco is relatively drought-tolerant once established. Most plants are short-lived, lasting only a season or two. Occasionally new plants will sprout from last year's old crowns, if the winter was relatively mild. If your plants don't reseed themselves you will have to replant each year.

Gathering tips: I like to use a pair of garden snippers or my nails to remove a few leaves from each plant that I will be collecting from. Revisit your patches every 3 or 4 weeks, as the plants will continue to produce leaves throughout the spring and summer. After plants have gone to seed, consider collecting some seed to replant in a new area or in your yard.

Yerba Santa

(*Eriodictyon californicum*)
Saints' Herbs, Mountain Balm

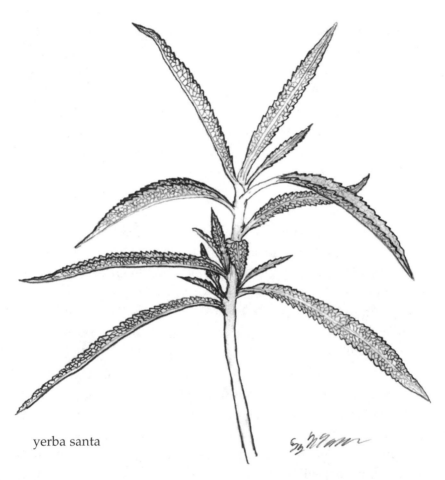

yerba santa

Yerba santa, or the saints' herb, is a California native, although it is found throughout much of the West. It is commonly called mountain balm by many California Natives. It is a traditional smoking and smudging herb.

Unlike mullein, yerba santa does not follow people's footsteps. The places yerba santa chooses to grow tend to have an ancient, Sacred feel about them. When people encroach on its territory by making roads or other construction, it responds by carrying on as best as it can. It tends to hold its own ground until the energy or the environment has changed drastically. When all the wildness is gone from a place, it is very rare to find yerba santa.

Burn or carry yerba santa to nurture and protect that which is ancient, Sacred, and wild within yourself. Use it when you need encouragement to hold your own ground and for courage when the time for retreat is at hand.

Yerba santa is one of my favorite herbs to burn as a tool to warm up trigger points on my feet and hands. If used very carefully, small bundles made of yerba santa can also be used to warm trigger points on the face and neck. Care must be taken not to set one's hair on fire. I use yerba santa in this way for relief of headache and muscle spasms.

Other uses: Yerba santa is used as a tea for coughs and fevers, and it is infused in oil for muscle and chest rubs. Salve made by infusing yerba santa in coconut oil is a superior remedy for dry skin and chapped lips.

Yerba santa plants, when in bloom, attract hummingbirds, as do mullein, wild tobacco, and some of the larger flowering monardas. A garden of herbs for burning will not only be delightfully fragrant—it will attract these bright and graceful visitors.

Growing tips: Yerba santa is a difficult plant to grow, because it seeks wild places. A site with good drainage, ideally on a slope, with barren rocky soil that is exposed to wind, rain and sun, would suit yerba santa's wild heart. Good drainage and full or nearly full sun is a must. A spot that will not be irrigated in summer once the young plants are established is also important if you want your yerba santa to be long lived.

Gathering tips: I collect yerba santa from large stands and only one sprig or a leaf or two from each plant. I first talk to the plant, listening for any special instructions it may offer me. When there are none I make sure the plant agrees to the use for which I am gathering.

If you live near where yerba santa grows, visit the patches you tend regularly through the summer. Study the growing tips and follow the branch back towards the trunk. There you will find what Grandmother called "ripe leaves." The green has begun to drain from these leaves; they have begun to get yellow or even dry around the edges. When asked, the bush will often release these leaves at the slightest brush of your hand.

These ripe leaves were my grandmother's favored ones to gather from yerba santa plants if they were going to be burned.

Sources

Purchasing Smudge Herbs

Some Native traditionalists frown on the idea of buying herbs for smudge. It is generally felt that you should prepare smudge yourself, or receive it as a gift or as part of a trade. This can be troublesome for urban Natives who may find that the only thing available for trade in their work-a-day lifestyle is money. Those Native people who spend time, money, and care producing smudge sticks for sale are often on the receiving end of ridicule and censorship by those who disapprove. Nonetheless, many urban Native people purchase smudge from health-food stores, herb and recovery shops, trading posts, or from vendors at powwows.

Herbs that are not gathered and prepared for smudge are not preferred, but if they are all that is available they are acceptable. When you get them home, place them on your altar or other special place. Invite the Spirit of the Herb to join you and guide you in your Sacred Work. Whether you speak to them silently through your heart or aloud, is up to you. Do whatever makes the process seem the most real. Use respect, kindness, and affection when addressing the Spirit of the Herb. Consider having the intention to form a long-lasting friendship and partnership.

CMC Company
PO Drawer 322
Avalon NJ 08202
(800) CMC-2780
(609) 861-3065 fax
web page: www.thecmccompany.com
Source for dried epazote leaves.

The Cooking Post
Pueblo of Santa Anna
2 Dove Road
Bernalillo NM 87004
email: info@cookingpost.com
Native American company that offers peppermint tea.

Esencial Dreams
70 Iris Lane
Canton NC 28716
(228) 648-4834
web page: www.esencialdreams.com
Native American company with a variety of resins, smudge sticks, juniper, and other herbs.

Forest Farm
900 Tetherow Rd.
Williams OR 97544-9599
(541) 846-7269
web page: www.forestfarm.com
This large mail-order nursery carries bayberry, cedar, incense cedar, juniper, and *Artemisia tridentata* plants. They have many varieties of pine, including Italian stone pine, lodgepole pine, several varieties of piñon, *Pinus contorta*, and ponderosa pine; many varieties of fir, including Douglas fir, balsam fir, and *Abies lasiocarpa*; and hemlock, including *Tsuga heterophylla*. The $5.00 fee for the catalog is well worth the price. Information about needle length, pitch levels, preferred habitat, and uses are given for many trees.

Las Pilitas Nursery
3232 Las Pilitas Road
Santa Margarita CA
(805) 438-5992 or (760) 749-5930
web page: www.laspilitas.com
email: bawilson@laspilitas.com

Look for artemisias, cedars, firs, incense cedar, juniper, mints, monarda, pine, sage, salvias, uva ursi, yerba santa. Catalog is $10.00, price list is free. Be sure to visit their web site. Although they are not up to date on Native uses of plants, the site is otherwise very informative.

Mountain Valley Growers
38325 Pepperweed Road
Squaw Valley CA 93675
(559) 338-2775
web page: www.mountainvalleygrowers.com
email: ice@mountainvalleygrowers.com
Source for sweet grass plants.

Native Seed/SEARCH
526 North 4th Ave.
Tucson AZ 85705-8450
web page: info@nativeseeds.org
This Native American company offers dried epazote leaves, seeds of several types of wild tobacco, and a few other herbs.

Richters Herbs
Goodwood
Ontario, LOC 1A0
Canada
(905) 640-6677
(905) 640-6641 fax
web page: www.richters.com
Seeds and plants of fennel, epazote, and *Artemisia cana.* Seeds and leaves of mints and monardas. Seeds, plants, and dried leaves of mugwort. Mullein seeds, plants, dried leaves, and dried flowers. Plants and dried leaves of uva ursi. Dried root and seeds of osha and lomation. Benzoin gum, frankincense, myrrh, and acacia resin as gum arabic. Wild tobacco seeds. Juniper berries.

Sioux Trading Post
415 Sixth Street
Rapid City SD 57701
(800) 456-3394
Native American company offers osha root, plants and dried leaves of uva ursi, as well as other roots and herbs.

Starwest Botanicals, Inc
11253 Trade Center Drive
Rancho Cordova CA 95742
(916) 853-9354
email: sales-w@starwestbotanicals.com
Wholesale dry herbs and herbal products.

Sweet Grass
51 Great Bar
Keshena WI 54185
web page: www.sweetgrass.com
email: info@sweetgrass.com
Native American company offering sweet grass braids.

Trinity Alps Botanicals
P.O. Box 196
Burnt Ranch CA 95527
(530) 629-3311
email: tab@pcweb.net
web page: trinityalpsbotanicals.com
This Native American business has dried California bay, incense cedar, fir, pine, mullein, yerba santa, and other herbs and herbal products.

Tsemeta Nursery
P.O. Box 368
Hoopa CA 95546-0368
(530) 625-4206
email: tsemeta@pcweb.net
This Native American tribal enterprise offers plants, dried herbs, and custom wildcrafting to wholesale buyers only.

About Herb Books and Web Sites

Any book, when compared to traditional teachings, is artificial and shallow. Books are alien concepts within the context of Native traditions and passing on teachings. I as a writer and you as a reader must keep this fact in mind.

As very young children we first begin to understand about words, reading, and writing. One of the first things we learn is about the permanence of print. If you write a sentence or two about the sunrise on a piece of paper, those words will stay the same. If you read them in spring or winter, if you read them in the river valley or on the mountain top, if you read them to an elder or to a child, the words on that paper are still the same.

When we write down information that is essentially a part of the oral tradition, it diminishes the information. Teaching about plants is like talking about the sunrise. That talk changes with the season, the place, and the people we speak to. When we teach about plant knowledge, what we say depends on many things. This knowledge is not fixed and permanent like words on a page. It is living and growing and changing as we live and grow and change.

I and other writers have fixed words on paper about our experiences with plants. These words can serve as hints to you. Read what several authors say about the herbs. This will broaden your perspective, in ways that reading only one author's words can never do.

For this purpose of broadening perspective, I have included text and web page references. Don't forget that all these words are fixed and narrow and that traditional knowledge about plants is broad and fluid. My hope is that reading about the plants in the books and on the web sites and comparing that information to this book will begin to open your mind to the complexities of having a relationship with the plants.

Very few of the references actually address burning the herbs. Not all of these books adequately address safety concerns.

As you read in the references and web pages about what other authors have written about these plants, you may find references to them being harmless, poisonous, and even European. Calling a medicine harmless is disrespectful. It disrespects the power of the plant's medicine. Calling medicine poisonous can poison us against our traditions and the healing offered us by the plants.

However, calling a Native medicine "European" and saying that we learned how to use it from the invaders is the greatest disrespect of all. It affects our wisdom traditions in much the same way that killing the buffalo affected many tribes' subsistence food traditions. Remember history when you read these kinds of statements about our medicines. Sift out the information that is useful to you. Speak with your elders. Listen to the plants.

One final caution on using the information you gain through research. You will find that many herbs were used for very different things by different tribes. If you cataloged all these uses, as some herb books and web sites do, you might think it was a good idea to use a single plant for many things.

Please remember that our ancestors did very little by accident. Plants occupied specific places in a tribe's or a particular grandmother's pharmacopoeia. This is for many reasons.

The chemical constituents of plants change from region to region depending on the environment, weather, soil, and the other plants and animals present. This can affect the plant's medicinal value and other actions. Many plants contain naturally occurring toxins in minute levels. Limiting our exposure to these natural toxins is an important consideration. Additionally, we must think of the pressure on plant populations and guard against overharvesting.

I want to encourage you to read all you can, but please, keep tradition in mind while you read.

USE YOUR LOCAL LIBRARY!

Most of the books on the following list are in my personal library. However, you do not need to buy each of these books to get a balanced perspective on using herbs for smudge. A visit to your local library will probably turn up at least a few of these titles.

Public and many college libraries have a system for borrowing books from other libraries. If you don't find the titles you are looking for, ask the librarian how to request a book from another library, or how to reserve a particular book in your name for when it's returned. This service is often free, however some libraries charge a small fee to cover postage and other costs.

Using this service will allow you to read out-of-print, hard to find, or expensive items. It will also allow you to review a book before you decide if you want to purchase it for your own collection.

Many public and college libraries have public computers you can use to access the internet. Some libraries require you to reserve a short block of time in advance, other libraries have computers available on a first-come-first-serve basis. Inquire at your local library about this service. If you have never used the internet before, you can also inquire about a class or a tutor to help you get comfortable accessing the world wide web.

In any event it is good to show up with a note pad and pencil, a computer disc, or a pocket full of change. Libraries usually charge a nominal fee for printing.

You don't need to have a large budget to explore literary knowledge on the subject of plant medicine.

The herbs I've shared are all long-time friends of mine. I also used the following books for botanical names, to jog my memory, or to give physical-world confirmation to what I knew from Spiritual sources.

Book List

The Audubon Society Pocket Guide—Familiar Trees of North America, Jerry F. Franklin (contributor). 1987, Knopf, ISBN 0394748514. (Good for botanical names and identification.)

Back to Eden, Jethro Kloss. Back to Eden Books, ISBN 0-940676-00-1. (Fennel, mugwort, mullein, uva ursi, yerba santa.)

School of Natural Healing, Dr. John R. Christopher. Bi World Publishing, 1996, ISBN 1879436019. (Epazote, mullein, myrrh, uva ursi, pennyroyal, peppermint, spearmint, horsemint, etc.)

Earth Medicine Earth Foods, Michael A. Weiner. Collier Books. (Juniper, sage.)

Encyclopedia of Herbs & Herbalism, edited by Malcom Stuart. Crescent Publishing, ISBN 0-517-353261. (Cautions are sometimes found in the medicinal action or other uses section and sometimes in their own section entitled "Cautions." Epazote listed as American wormseed, myrrh, benzoin, camphor, and wild tobacco.)

An Ethnobiology Source Book, The Uses of Plants and Animals by American Indians, edited with an introduction by Richard Ford. Garland Publishing, 1986, ISBN 0-8240-5894-1. (Part of a 20-volume series. This is the book containing the reference on California bay. This book is very informative, but it is difficult to use and even harder to find. Bayberry, juniper, various resins and gums, osha, and sage.)

The Healing Herbs, Michael Castleman. Rodale Books, ISBN 087857-934-6. (Cautionary information is listed for each herb in a section called "The Safety Factor." Bayberry.)

Herbs, An Illustrated Encyclopedia, Kathy Keville. Friedman/Fairfax, ISBN 1-56799-065-7. (Cautions are listed in a section called "Considerations" for those herbs necessary. Fennel.)

Herbs & Things, Jeanne Rose. Grosset & Dunlap, ISBN 0448-01139-5. (Good information on safety and side effects of herbs. Uses a symbol system, no in-depth specific information. Mugwort, myrrh, and yerba santa. Epazote is listed as Jerusalem oak; European sweet grass is listed as vernal grass.)

Herbal Home Remedy Book, Joyce Wardell. Storey Publishing, ISBN 1-58017-016-1. (Mullein.)

Kashaya Pomo Plants, Jeanine Goodrich, Claudia Lawson, Vana Parrish Lawson. Heyday Books, ISBN 0-930588-86-X. (Wild tobacco, mugwort, yerba santa.)

Magic and Medicine of Plants, edited and published by Readers' Digest. ISBN 0-89577-221-3. (Very easy-to-use information that lets you know at a glance if there are cautions for each plant covered. Epazote listed as wormseed.)

Montana Native Plants and Early Peoples, Jeff Hart. Montana Historical Society Press, 1996, ISBN 0-917298-29-2. (Sweet grass and root.)

Medicinal Plants of The Mountain West, Michael Moore. Museum of New Mexico Press, ISBN 0-89013-104-X. (Cautions are included in "Medicinal Use" sections for each herb. Juniper, osha root, sage, wild tobacco, and yerba santa.)

Native American Ethnobotany, Daniel A. Moerman. Timberpress Inc., 1998, ISBN 0-88192-453-9. (Root.)

Native Plants Native Healing, Tis Mal Crow. Native Voices, 2001, ISBN 1-57067-105-2. (Gathering information.)

Natural Health, Natural Healing, Andrew Weil M.D. Houghton Mifflin, ISBN 0-395-58122-2. (Peppermint, mullein, uva ursi.)

The New Age Herbalist, Richard Maybey. Collier Books, ISBN 0-02-063350-5. (Some cautionary information is listed, but much that should be is left out. However, this is a great book in many other ways. Bayberry.)

New Western Garden Book. Sunset, ISBN 376-03890-X. (Cedar, juniper, bayberry, good for botanical names.)

Ornamental Trees, Evelyn Maino and Frances Howard. University of California Press, ISBN 0-520-00795-6. (Cedar, juniper.)

Pacific Coastal Wildlife Region, Charles Yocum and Ray Dasmann. Naturegraph Publishers. (California bay is listed as California laurel.)

Plants of the Pacific Northwest Coast, Jim Pojar and Andy Mackinnon. Lone Pine Publishing, 1994, ISBN 1-55105-040-4. (Sweet grass.)

Plants of Power, Alfred Savinelli. Native Voices, 2002, ISBN 1-57067-130-3. (Incense cedar, juniper, mugwort, osha, piñon pine, white sage, desert sage, sweet grass, ceremonial tobacco, yerba santa.)

Temalpakh, Cahuilla Indian Knowledge and Usage of Plants, Lowell John Bean and Katherine Siva Saubel. Malki Museum Press, ISBN 0-939-046-24-5. (Wild tobacco, cedar, juniper, sage, and California bay listed as mountain laurel.)

The Way of Herbs, Michael Tierra, C.A., N.D. Orenda, ISBN 0-913300-43-8. (Fennel, peppermint, spearmint, mugwort, uva ursi.)

Smudge on the Web

Some of these web sites may expire or change. If you do not find the information you are looking for, I have found the best way to search is usually by using the botanical name of the plant. If you get too many listings to sift through, use the botanical name and a slash and list the specific information you want. Here is an example:

Umbellularia californica/Native uses

If you still do not find the information you want, try the common name or reword the type of information you want. Here is another example:

California bay/American Indian uses

Bayberry

More information on bayberry as well as color photos can be found on the following web sites.

For *Myrica californica* see:

http://www.hortpix.com/pc2834.htm

For *Myrica cerifera* see:

http://www.herbs2stopsmoking.com/herbdesc/2bayberr.htm

For *Myrica pennsylvania* see:

http://wadell.ci-manchester.ct.us/id-bayberry.htm1

California bay, *Umbellularia californica*

This site has links to lots of information and a list of references for even more information:

http://www.fs.fed.us/database/feis/plants/tree/umbcal/

This site takes a while to load, but if you are patient you can scroll down to a photo of a fairly young cultivated tree:

http://www.hortpix.com/pc4362.htm

For a picture of immature "peppernuts" check out this site:

http://www.botgard.ucla.edu/html/MEMBGNewsletter/Volume3number4/a0801tx.html

Photos of flowers and leaves plus links to photos of mature "pepper-nuts," old bark, and young bark. This is very cool for identification purposes!

http://www.biologie.uniulm.de/systax/dendrologie/Umbecaliflw.htm

Outline of a mature tree:

http://www.pennine.demon.co.uk/Arboretum/Umca.htm

Photo of a stand of wild trees, as they typically appear in coastal environments:

http://www.callutheran.edu/wf/chap/flowers/fwr-681.htm

Cedar, *Libocedrus decurrens* (Incense Cedar):

Good close-up picture of leaves and pods:

http://www.iastate.edu/~bot356/species/species/k_oSpecic/LiboDecu.html

Picture of incense cedar tree in wild:

http://www.laspilitas.com/plants/386.htm

Picture of young cultivated tree:

http://www.dipbot.unict.it/orto/0627-1.html

More information, no pictures:

http://www.na.fs.fed.us/spfo/pubs/silvics_manual/Volume_1/libocedrus/decurrens.htm

Chamaecyparis lawsoniana (Port-Orford-Cedar):

Information and scroll down for picture of cultivated tree:

http://bluehen.ags.udel.edu/gopherdata2/.conifers/.descriptions/c_lawsoniana.html

Photo of baby tree showing leaf structure:

http://bluehen.ags.udel.edu/gopherdata2/.conifers/.descriptions/c_lawsoniana.html

Thuja plicata (Western Red Cedar):

Information and picture of trunk of mature tree:
http://www.mastergardenproducts.com/redcedar.htm

Picture of mature wild trees:
http://www.wsu.edu/~wsherb/images/Cupressaceae/thuja.html

Scroll down for a drawing of a sprig and close-up of leaves:
http://www.nearctica.com/trees/conifer/cupress/Tplica.htm

Juniperus scopulorum:

This site has links to more information:
http://www.fs.fed.us/database/feis/plants/tree/junsco/

Nice close-up photo of a sprig with berries:
http://classes.hortla.wsu.edu/hort232/list3/
Juniperus_scopulorum.html

Scroll down on this site for photos of *Juniperus scopulorum* in the home landscape:
http://www.mpelectric.com/treebook/fact41.html

Pictures of *Juniperus scopulorum* growing in the wild:
http://biology.usgs.gov/npsveg/scbl/pinjun.html

Juniperus occidentalis:

Information:
http://www.na.fs.fed.us/spfo/pubs/silvics_manual/Volume_1/
juniperus/occidentalis.htm

Picture of a mature wild tree in its natural habitat:
http://ag.arizona.edu/classes/ram382/plntpix/juoc.html

Picture of a fairly mature cultivated specimen of *Juniperus occidentalis*:
http://www.csu.org/cgibin/xeri/Xeriinclude?Xeridetail?PIS-jot

Close-ups of branches, leaves, and berries:
http://www.orst.edu/instruct/for241/con/spp/junspp.html

Fennel

Photo of mature wild plant in full bloom:
http://www.bahiker.com/pictures/southbay/mcnee/081800/websize/013fennel.jpg

Photos of young cultivated plants with information on growing:
http://melanys.tripod.com/Fennel.htm

Medicinal information on fennel:
http://www.bagelhole.org/article.php/Health/57/

Great picture of fennel leaves and a nice article on uses:
http://www.sallys-place.com/food/columns/gilbert/fennel.htm

Mint

Good information on growing a variety of mint species:
http://www.botany.com/mentha.html

List of mint species with links to photos and distribution maps:
http://www.csdl.tamu.edu/FLORA/cgi/ruled_html_query?colldir
=kartesz%2Fmgdata&collname=bonap98&query=Mentha

Information on monardas, scroll down for more species and pictures:
http://www.ibiblio.org/herbmed/eclectic/kings/monarda.html

More information on monarda with links to information on other mints:
http://www.botanical.com/botanical/mgmh/b/bergam32.html

Mugwort

Nice close-up pictures of leaves and flowers as well as some information on the chemistry and etymology of mugwort. Use arrows on right of page to scroll down to second picture:
http://wwwang.kfunigraz.ac.at/~katzer/engl/generic_frame.html?
Arte_vul.html

This site tells about the medicinal benefits of mugwort from a European perspective:

http://www.botanical.com/botanical/mgmh/m/mugwor61.html

(Mugwort, cont.)

This site explores the dream stimulation aspects of mugwort and discusses the fact that it should not be used in pregnancy.
http://home.teleport.com/~howieb/treats/mugwort.html

More mugwort pictures:
http://www.ecnca.org/Plants/Information/mugwort.htm

Mullein

This site has great pictures and information on mullein from a European perspective:
http://altnature.com/gallery/mullein.htm

Scroll down on this site for information on mullein being used in many cultures to ward off evil spirits:
http://www.geocities.com/nutriflip/Naturopathy/Mullein.html

Information on growing mullein:
http://www.mofga.org/mofgs997.html

Scroll down on this page for another Native view on mullein:
http://www.cherokee.org/TribalGovernment/
SR2000HistCulturePage.asp?ID=2

Pine, Fir, and Hemlock

Everything you ever wanted to know about piñon pine can be found on this site:
http://www.fs.fed.us/database/feis/plants/tree/pinon/
value_and_use.html

This site has a distribution map, pictures, and some information for lodge pole pine:
http://www.treeguide.com/nn/Species.asp?Region
=NorthAmerican&SpeciesID=694

Scroll down on this page for a list of tree names, and click on the botanical name for pictures, links, and lots of information:
http://www.nearctica.com/trees/conifer/bylist.htm

Information on Native evergreens in the home landscape:
http://www.colostate.edu/Depts/CoopExt/4DMG/Trees/
natever.htm

Resins

List of trees, many have uses listed for their pitch:
http://interactive.usask.ca/skinteractive/modules/forestry/
industry/types_softwood.html

Lots of information and links on the history and uses of frankincense:
http://www.botanical.com/botanical/mgmh/f/franki31.html

The history and chemical composition of myrrh are:
http://www.chem.ox.ac.uk/mom/myrrh/myrrh2.html

This site gives photos, information, and links to a number of trees
whose resins are used in a variety of ways:
http://waynesword.palomar.edu/ecoph22.html

A brief history of incense is given on this site, including information
on resins:
http://www.incense-wholesale.com/herbal/story.html

How to make incense from gum arabic and various resins. It also
gives some information on beliefs about incense from Japanese legends:
http://www.lesliekenton.com/activebar/updates/new_this_week/
archives/herb16.htm

Root

Scroll down for pictures and some information on *Ligusticum porteri*:
http://www.swcoloradowildflowers.com/White%20Enlarged%20P
hoto%20Pages/heracleum%20sphondylium.htm

Medicinal information on *Ligusticum porteri* is available on this site;
http://www.backcountryrangers.com/edibles/
plantssoloframe.html?LOMATIUM.html

Medicinal information on *Lomatium dissectum* is available at this
site:
http://www.healthwell.com/healthnotes/Herb/Lomatium.cfm

Sage, Desert, *Artemisia tridentata*

Distribution map:
http://www.ibiblio.org/pub/academic/medicine/alternative-healthcare/herbalmedicine/SWSBM/Maps/Artemisia_tridentata.gif

Picture and some medicinal information:
http://vitalvillage.net/nmc/nmc-pages/desertsage.htm

Picture and scientific information on *Artemisia tridentata*:
http://www.usask.ca/agriculture/plantsci/classes/range/artemisiatriden.html

Scroll down for a chart showing Native use of various artemisias, including *Artemisia tridentata*. Scroll farther for a list of books that contain information on Native uses of plants:
http://www.geocities.com/Athens/Olympus/6581/goddessgarden9.html

Sweet Grass

Keep scrolling for a drawing of plant, pictures of sweet grass braids and sweet grass baskets, lots of information including native uses and links:
http://www.nativetech.org/plants/sweetgrass.html

Scroll down for lots of growing information and pictures of a single plant and a nice stand of cultivated plants:
http://www.ecoseeds.com/sweetgrass.html

Photos of beautiful Native-made sweet grass baskets:
http://www.savageart.com/basket.html

This site lists a small amount of medicinal and other information on sweet grass with links to pages listing many references containing information on sweet grass:
http://www.fs.fed.us/database/feis/plants/graminoid/hieodo/value_and_use.html

Uva Ursi

This site has information on medicinal uses:
http://www.botanical.com/botanical/mgmh/b/bearbe22.html

Photos showing flowers, leaves, and berries:
http://www.ct-botanical-society.org/galleries/
arctostaphylosuva-.html

Photo showing low-growing, ground-hugging habit of plant:
http://www.erowid.org/herbs/show_image.php3?image=uvaursi/
images/archive/arctostaphylos_uvaursi2.jpg

Lots of information including a picture and some information on Native uses of uva ursi:
http://www.rook.org/earl/bwca/nature/shrubs/arctouvaursi.html

Wild Tobacco

Here is a very interesting scientific article about plant communication between sage brush and wild tobacco:
http://www.ice.mpg.de/departments/Ecol/publications%20Ian/
karban%20baldwin%20baxter%20communication%20
oecologia%202000.pdf

Scientific article on wild tobacco communicating with predator insects, includes a photo of a wild tobacco plant:
http://www.sciam.com/news/031601/4.html

Scroll down for some history on tobacco and nicotine:
http://micro.magnet.fsu.edu/moviegallery/chemicalcrystals/
nicotine/56k/nicotine07.html

Picture of wild tobacco:
http://www.northcountrytrail.org/pwf/images/wildtobacco1.JPG

Yerba Santa

This site has a distribution map, medicinal information, and pictures of the plants in flower:
http://www.ibiblio.org/london/alternativehealthcare/Southwest-
School-of-Botanical-Medicine/FOLIOS/YerbaFol.pdf

(Yerba Santa, cont.)

This site has lots of links (double click), if you scroll down you will also find information on yerba santa's chemical constituents:

http://www.herbmed.org/herbs/Eriodictyon_YerbaSanta.htm#folk

Effect of range-land fire on yerba santa:

http://www.fs.fed.us/database/feis/plants/shrub/erical/fire_effects.html

Yerba santa and high tech skin care:

http://www.cosmetic-lasersurg.com/yerba.htm

About
Harvest McCampbell

Harvest McCampbell is a highly respected Native American herbalist, author, and educator. She is also a gifted artist and storyteller. She has been touching and healing the hearts of the young and old for twenty years with her knowledge, skill, and experience. Her writings and teachings are known throughout the West.

Harvest was born Iroquois Onondaga Oswegatchie, Bear Clan. She became skilled in the ways of the Old Ones as a young girl through the teachings of her Native American grandmother, who taught her to identify, gather, and process herbs for medicine and ceremony. She grew up eating wild plant foods and preparing medicines from plants she skillfully processed. From the beginning, she was enveloped in the spirit and traditions of Native culture. After the passing of her grandmother, Harvest continued her tutelage under several prominent herbologists and became a Certified Herbalist and U.C. Master Gardener.

Aside from being one of the most highly skilled Native American herbalists today, Harvest is equally respected for her teaching and sharing of the Old Ways with others. She taught Ethnobotany at DQ University, the only tribal college in California. In addition, she has been teaching herb classes throughout central and northern California for over 20 years, through which she has passed on her knowledge of herb gathering, processing, and usage, as well as plant identification. Her previously published books on Native herbs have sold thousands of copies. She is also an accomplished poet and ceramic artist with several awards for her poetry and ceramics. Harvest has worked closely with the Indian community for many years and is especially devoted to promoting literacy among the Indian children on the reservation where she now resides.

From a place of quiet solitude nestled in the mountains, Harvest now shares her knowledge and experience with herbs mainly through her writings. She has pulled back from her public life of teaching to live in a Native community, where she works closely with the local elders as she studies in her classroom that is Mother Earth. Harvest continues to share this knowledge through her writings to "help mend the damage done to the web of creation."

In this book, Harvest teaches us to have respect for the power of the healing herbs. She teaches us how to gather herbs in a Sacred Way by telling us how she gathers from her "special wild places." This book tells the story of Harvest's life and how she has come to live at one with the earth through the traditional methods of gathering, replanting, giving thanks, and doctoring those in need. For Harvest, learning about tradition is a lifetime journey that will never cease, and she implores us to seek out our own elders today so that we may keep our own traditions alive.

Renee Shahrokh
Lori Fox-Rigney

Index

prayer sticks 85
Prayer, Women's 18
pregnancy 36, 50-51, 61, 65, 66,
        91, 116

R

Rainbow Woman 18
recovery 8, 101
religious freedom 8
reservations, Indian 25, 122
resin 79-81, 102, 109, 117
respiratory distress 35
rheumatism 79
ritual 13, 33, 34, 46, 65
ritual bath 29
root 27, 83, 84, 104, 110

S

Sacred Beings 93
sacred bundles 12
Sacred Circle 16
Sacred herbs 13, 21
Sacred practice 21
sacred rattles 12
sacred spiral 12, 30
Sacred valley 16
Sacred Way 33, 43, 47, 85, 122
Sacred Work 101
sage 85-89, 103, 109-111, 119
        bark 86
        brush 85
        black 85
        blue 85
        desert 47, 85-86, 111, 118
        silver 85
        white 85, 111
saints' herb 95
salvia 85, 103
sap 75, 79, 80, 81
scabies 93
sinus infection 80

Sky World 23, 30
sore throat 40, 80, 89
spearmint 109, 111
spider bites 45
Spirit Beings 23
Spirit helpers 47
Spirit of the Herb 101
spirochetosis 93
spruce 73, 79-80
stomachache 40, 61, 62, 89
suffering 14, 15, 16, 36
Sun Dance 16
sweat lodge 15, 27, 29, 39, 43, 49,
        52, 65, 76, 83
sweet fern 39
sweet gale 39
sweet grass 21, 23, 39, 89, 90,
        103-104, 110-111, 118
sweet gum 79

T

Taxus brevifolia 49
tea
        balsam fir 80
        bayberry 40
        epazote 55
        fennel 60
        fir 75, 76
        incense cedar 49
        juniper 51
        mint 61, 62, 63
        monarda 61
        mullein 69, 70
        osha 83
        peppermint 102
        pine bark 73
        ritual 33
        sage 85
        sweet grass 89
        tobacco 93, 94
        uva ursi 91
        yerba santa 96

☞ Native Voices

tribal legends, medicine, arts & crafts,
history, life experiences, spirituality

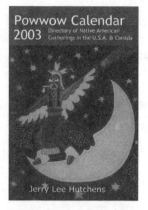

Powwow Calendar 2003
comp. by Jerry Lee Hutchens
1-57067-132-X $9.95

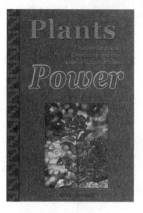

Plants of Power
Alfred Savinelli
1-57067-130-3 $9.95

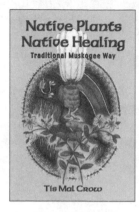

Native Plants, Native Healing
Tis Mal Crow
1-57067-105-2 $12.95

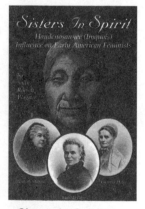

Sisters in Spirit
Sally Roesch Wagner
1-57067-121-4 $9.95

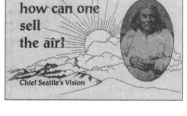

How Can One Sell the Air?
ed. by Eli Gifford & Michael Cook
0-913990-48-5 $7.95

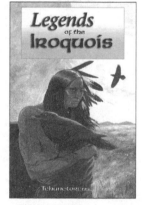

Legends of the Iroquois
Tehanetorens
1-57067-056-0 $9.95

Purchase these Native titles from your local bookstore, or you can buy them directly from:

Book Publishing Company
P.O. Box 99
Summertown, TN 38483
1-800-695-2241

Please include $3.95 per book for shipping and handling.

To find your Native books and products online, visit:
www.nativevoices.com